Learning Music Through Rhythm

By MARGUERITE V. HOOD

Associate Professor of Music, University of Michigan

Ann Arbor, Michigan

and E. J. SCHULTZ

University of Oklahoma, Norman, Oklahoma

GREENWOOD PRESS, PUBLISHERS
WESTPORT, CONNECTICUT

The Library of Congress has catalogued this publication as follows:

Library of Congress Cataloging in Publication Data

Hood, Marguerite Vivian.
   Learning music through rhythm.

   Bibliography: p.
   1. Musico--callisthenics. I. Schultz, Ernest
John, joint author. I. Title.
[MT948.H69 1972]   780'.77   74-138151
ISBN 0-8371-5608-4

Acknowledgments

The authors wish to thank Miss Helen S. Leavitt for the wise counsel and valuable service which she has given to them in the preparation of this book.

Acknowledgment is due also for "Tomorrow" from SPANISH-AMERICAN FOLK SONGS, used by courtesy of the author, Miss Eleanor Hague, and the American Folklore Society; for "Danish Reel" from THE RHYTHMS OF CHILDHOOD by Caroline Crawford and Elizabeth Rose Fogg, copyright 1915 by A. S. Barnes and Company; for "Little Man in a Fix" from RING DANCES AND SINGING GAMES by Mary Wood Hinman, copyright 1930 by A. S. Barnes and Company; for "John Pirulera" compiled by Workers of the Writers' Program, Music Program and Art Program of the Work Projects Administration in the State of New Mexico, SPANISH-AMERICAN SONG AND GAME BOOK, A. S. Barnes and Company, New York, 1942; for "Four in a Boat" by courtesy of the Cooperative Recreation Service, Delaware, Ohio; for "The Cricket" poem by Clinton Scollard, used by permission of Jessie B. Rittenhouse; for "Rock-a-by" poem by J. G. Holland, used by permission of Charles Scribner's Sons; for "The Elephant" from PROMENADE ALL, compiled and published by Janet E. Tobitt; for "Jack be Nimble" by Lily Strickland from Frost's ORIENTAL AND CHARACTER DANCES, used by permission of A. S. Barnes and Company; to the editors of THE WORLD OF MUSIC and to Ginn and Company for permission to use in this book many songs and piano selections which have added so much to its enrichment.

Contents

CONTENTS

CONTENTS

Introduction

Rhythm is movement; it is the interpretation of the musical phrase and measure. This interpretation is expressed most appropriately by children through physical response. Before pupils can make suitable responses they must learn to listen in order that they may feel the rhythm and express their feeling in some satisfactory way. Through much experience in physical response, rhythmic consciousness is developed.

There was a time when educators felt that a purely intellectual approach to the reading of various rhythmic patterns was the only satisfactory method. These teachers thought that knowledge of note values based on mathematics would insure a correct interpretation of different rhythmic combinations. But even though a sixteenth note has one-fourth the value of a quarter note, and though it is possible to determine the number of beats in a measure and the various groupings of notes for each beat, this information alone will be likely to lead to a mechanical rendition. To secure an interpretation with emotional appeal it is necessary that the pupil be led to sense the rhythm. Various combinations and arrangements of notes should set up certain _feeling_ responses in his psycho-physical system.

People who read rhythmic notation will find it impossible to scan the notation of rhythmic patterns without feeling a physical, muscular reaction of some sort. It is the purpose of the activities outlined in this book to develop within children appropriate feeling responses to rhythms heard, and to their corresponding symbols. After children have experienced these rhythmic activities, they will read rhythmic notation from a _feeling_ standpoint. They will look at notes of various kinds and will be able to sing or play them correctly as to rhythm because they can feel the movement of the notes. This feeling is a result of their experience of response through stepping, walking, skipping, running, and many other movements.

Composers first feel and create rhythms and then determine the appropriate symbols for recording them. In similar manner, experience with various rhythms should precede the presentation of the symbols (notes, rests, measure bars, signatures, etc.) used to record the rhythmic patterns. To expect children to read notations they have not experienced and do not feel is neither psychologically nor pedagogically sound.

The child who is rhythmically weak is in as unfortunate a condition musically as one who is weak tonally but has a good sense of rhythm. Most musical instruments will produce pitch quite faithfully if the correct key is struck, the right hole covered, or the proper valve used; but no instrument will furnish the rhythmic drive for the performer. This orderly accent and grouping of tones must be felt by the player and be furnished by him; the instrument cannot help him. Therefore it is

INTRODUCTION

quite important that teachers, especially in the lower grades, take not only tonal inventory of their classes (discover the independent, the dependent, and the non-singers), but also take a rhythmic inventory of their pupils; discover those who re-spond readily to rhythmic accents, those whose attempts are hesitant, and those who are totally unable to respond satisfactorily.

Those children who do not respond appropriately to strongly rhythmic music need as much help as those who cannot match tones or carry a tune. Too often the nonrhythmic child is left undiscovered and neglected. It is hoped that teachers will use the activities which are suggested on the following pages in helping children to respond joyously to the beauties of rhythm in music.

Some forms of training the rhythmic sense which have been used in the past have been too elaborate and complicated for many teachers and have been too time-consuming in view of the limited number of minutes allotted to music. Some music educators have expressed the feeling that the training of the rhythmic sense is a part of physical training and properly belongs under the direction of the physical education teacher. There is a germ of plausibility in this viewpoint; but the ex-periences described on the succeeding pages are designed primarily to be of the greatest aid in the building of musical understanding and the development of music-reading ability, rather than the development of the physique, bodily grace, and mus-cular control. A certain amount of overlapping is not undesirable, however, if we incline toward the educational philosophy of integration.

It will be found that the activities in this course not only develop the rhythmic sense and the ability to read rhythmic notation, but are invaluable in cultivating the habit of listening to music—and listening all of the time. Pupils cannot perform these activities well if they are not listening to "what the music tells them to do." There is no better method of developing the power of aural attention than participation in experiences similar to those included in this book.

Rhythmic experiences supply the physical activities which are essential to every well-planned music lesson. Little children should not be expected to sit quietly in their seats for an entire recitation. The music period ought to be a time for joyous activity—the bright spot of the day; and any music period which is not enjoyed by the pupils and the teacher may be considered a failure. Children thor-oughly enjoy rhythmic activity, whereas they do not enjoy formal drill on the math-ematical values of notes and rests. However, enjoyment alone is not the only jus-tification; an activity should be educationally purposeful as well. It is believed that such activities as are suggested in the following pages fulfill both of these qual-ifications.

Notes and Suggestions for Teachers

1. It is suggested that the experiences of Chapters I to XIII be allocated to the primary grades, and that all of the chapters be covered by the end of the pupil's sixth year of school or before he completes all his required general music. Many of the experiences suggested for primary grade children (such as creative work, feeling for phrases, response to accent, and response to and reading of phrase rhythms) should be continued in the upper grades.

2. The order of the activities of this course need not be strictly followed in all situations. It is simply suggested as a successful, workable sequence. Any teacher using this book should present these experiences in the order best suited to her group. The important thing is for the pupil to experience all the phases of the course during his training in music.

3. The teacher need not feel that she should use every activity suggested in each chapter. Instead, she ought to select those which she can most effectively use. An abundance of suggestions is given in this book in order that the teacher may have a large number from which to make a selection.

4. The so-called "natural" rhythms (walking, running, skipping) are stressed because these rhythms correlate definitely with music notation. Rhythms used for purposes of imitation, such as rocking a cradle, flying like butterflies, dancing like fairies, walking like elephants, hopping like a rabbit or a kangaroo, or stealthily creeping like a goblin, have their place in the lesson where perception of mood, free movement, interpretation, and dramatization are emphasized rather than in the lesson where the attention is focused on rhythmic discrimination and rhythmic notation.

5. In the intermediate grades pupils may not derive the same enjoyment from stepping, running, and skipping as they did in the earlier grades. When such a condition exists, other activities, such as singing, sensing the meter and phrases of songs, and playing rhythmic patterns on instruments may be emphasized. However, reference to certain notes as "running," "skipping," "walking," "one-beat," and "two-beat" tones may be continued profitably, even in the upper grades, as well as quarter, half, and other different kinds of notes.

6. One purpose of the activities suggested in this book is to build rhythm vocabularies for the ear and eye through physical activity. Although tonal vocabularies are essential and the building of these vocabularies should be carried on with the rhythmic activities in the appropriate grades, no attempt is made in the succeeding pages to give suggestions for tonal vocabulary development.

7. The experiences outlined in this book prepare pupils as definitely for read-

ing instrumental music as for reading vocal music. Therefore it is essential that beginning with Chapter VIII not only vocal notations be used but instrumental notations as well; id est, the pupil should see not only ♪ ♪ ♪ ♪ and ♩ ♩ ♩ ♩. but also ♫,♫♫,♫ and ♫♫♫; not only ♪. ♪ and ♪. ♪♪. ♪ but ♩. ♩♩. ♩ and ♫♫ as well. Since instrumental class instruction is begun in many schools in the fifth grade, it is important that all of the phases of the first twelve steps be thoroughly mastered in the first four grades. The introduction stresses the relatively greater importance of rhythmic vocabulary (as compared to tonal vocabulary) for the instrumentalist (p.v). The teacher should realize that rhythmic sense-training should be emphasized, not only in order that the pupil may read <u>songs</u> with correct rhythm but also because it is of vital importance in instrumental work as well.

8. The teacher may use the piano or phonograph records when they are available. Some teachers can improvise at the piano, but in any case the music should be carefully selected and the specific rhythmic pattern clearly defined. It will be advantageous if the teacher can memorize the compositions which she plays so that she will be free to watch the pupils in their response and thus obtain a better idea of their natural tempi. Some examples of improvisations are found in this book which the teacher may find useful. However, these should not be used exclusively, for each teacher should be privileged to either improvise or choose other music which follows the patterns of the examples suggested.

9. With each musical example the correct tempo is indicated. Conditions in some classes may make it advisable to modify the rate of speed which is suggested, but the teacher should have sound and justifiable cause for any deviation. In every instance the natural tempo of the children should be discovered and used. Children's legs are shorter than those of an adult; therefore the natural tempo for an adult, whether walking or running, should not be used.

10. The activities herein suggested provide a wealth of opportunities for creative expression. Children like to make up their own responses to mood, to phrases, and to accent in music. After learning one or two folk dances or rhythm-band numbers by rote, the pupils should be encouraged to invent dance steps and to suggest rhythm-band orchestrations of their own.

In Grades One and Two children enjoy making up little sentence songs and tunes. With experience and with help from the teacher as needed, they gradually progress to making up tunes to two-line poems or couplets, and then four-line poems. Chapter Thirteen suggests in detail a plan for the writing of original tunes. This is a very important experience, and should be emphasized as soon as the pupils are sufficiently prepared. In creative activity the teacher may be tempted to keep the children's original melodies tonally and rhythmically simple in order that they may sing them with syllables and be able to write pitches as well as the phrase rhythms. It is recommended strongly that the teacher guard against this practice, and that the tunes created by the children be recorded faithfully, regardless of tonal or rhythmic difficulty. The pupils should write as much of their original music as they can, and the teacher should supply the rest. At all times original work should be kept original, even though the children's creations do not follow the problems in the grade outlines of our courses of study.

11. Individual work should not be neglected in rhythmic development. Each child should have an opportunity to experience rhythm <u>alone</u> at least once a week if it is at all possible. Very often in both vocal and rhythmic activities the individual is lost in the group, and surprising facts concerning individual pupils are revealed when they perform alone. Developing a rhythmic sense in the child who possesses little or none may be a slow process, even as the correction and elimination of "nonsingers" may take a year or more. Too much class time should not be given to the individual pupil, but his special needs should not be neglected.

12. Rhythm instruments provide a valuable medium of rhythmic sense-training and should be used when time permits. This training of the rhythmic sense is especially valuable in Chapters I, IV, VII, IX, and XII. While children enjoy the rhythm band very much, its use at all times should be purposeful from a music-education standpoint.

13. The songs and music suggested as preparatory material in connection with the various steps in this course should be learned well in advance of the time they are to be used, in order that the pupils may be thoroughly familiar with them.

14. Children must learn to feel rhythm through their <u>large</u> muscles if they are to sense the beauty of music. They must not be cramped or inhibited in any way. Therefore the beginning of rhythmic experience is greatly handicapped unless there is a large room available. Physical freedom is important, and children who can have their rhythmic experience in an open space not crowded with furniture are indeed fortunate. This cannot always be arranged, but in some situations it is possible to use the open halls in the school for such activities, and whenever the teacher can secure a place where the conditions are satisfactory she will find that the rhythmic experience becomes natural, spontaneous, and vital in a brief time.

LEARNING MUSIC THROUGH RHYTHM

Chapter I
First Experiences with Rhythm

The first and most natural rhythmic response for anyone, whether child or adult, is a simple, free movement made to the underlying rhythmic swing of music. Before a real study of rhythm and rhythmic patterns can begin successfully, it is necessary for a person to <u>feel</u> this steady <u>swing</u> in the music he hears and allow his muscles to respond to it spontaneously.

In this chapter the activities provide a variety of experiences for children of different ages which will help them in developing this ability to respond to rhythm or, in popular phraseology, to "keep time to the music." These experiences include action songs, free rhythmic activity with instrumental music, the use of rhythm instruments, and folk games and dances.

1. ACTION SONGS

Action or motion songs in which the accompanying movements are large, free, and simple, are ideal for early experience with rhythm. In some cases the motions are suggested by the words of the song; at other times they are simply movements which fit the rhythmic pattern of the music.

Row, Row, Row Your Boat	Did You Ever See a Lassie?
Soldier Boy	Bean Porridge Hot
We'll All Clap Hands Together	John Pirulero

are typical examples of action songs which may be used at various grade levels.

A. GENERAL SUGGESTIONS

It is usually best to wait until the children know the song thoroughly and can sing it well before introducing the rhythmic action. Once the action is suggested it becomes the center of interest, and from then on it is difficult to make any improvement in the singing of words and music.

It is important that the teacher keep in mind the purpose of these songs, namely, to develop ability to feel the rhythm of the music, and to respond to it through physical movement. Motions should not be inserted casually or vaguely at intervals. They should fit themselves to the rhythmic swing of the song and express it definitely.

1

The children who find it difficult to respond accurately to the rhythmic pattern of the song should participate often with those who have a strong feeling for the rhythm and respond correctly. A child who is weak in his response to rhythm needs a great deal of this type of experience. It is easy and enjoyable, and will teach him to relax and gain control of his muscles so that he can follow the steadily recurring pulsations in the music. The acquisition of such control will result in a positive improvement in the poise and self-assurance of the pupil.

Many teachers object to action songs because they believe that the strenuous movement required interferes with good tone production. This is frequently true. Therefore it is suggested that for such songs the class be divided; one half of the group will sing the song, the other half will express the "action" or rhythmic movement.

B. PROCEDURE

Row, Row, Row Your Boat

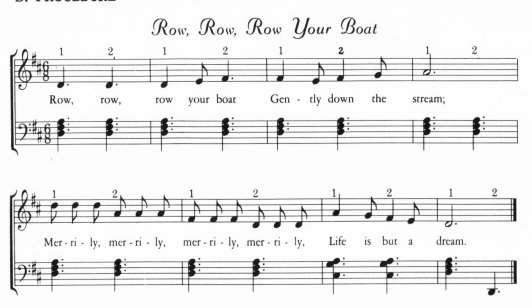

Because of these first rhythmic activities this song, which is often sung as a round, is learned here by rote as a unison song. In order to sing it with the right tempo, two rather than six beats should be used in each measure.

When the song is familiar, as half of the class sing the song, those who are to express the rhythmic action sit in their seats and pretend that they are rowing a boat, with an oar in each hand. With bodies bent slightly forward, they pull backward on the oars on the "1" marked in each measure of the music. On "2" the hands are pushed forward again so as to be ready for the next "1."

A reasonable amount of movement of the whole body should accompany this rowing motion. Some children may be inclined to use a vigorous bodily motion as the hands move backward and forward. Their responses will become more relaxed and natural if they are cautioned to row smoothly and easily, in order to save their energy for a long trip. Perhaps they will enjoy choosing a coxswain who sits facing them, either on the front desk or table, and counts the stroke just as is done for a racing boat crew.

Soldier Boy

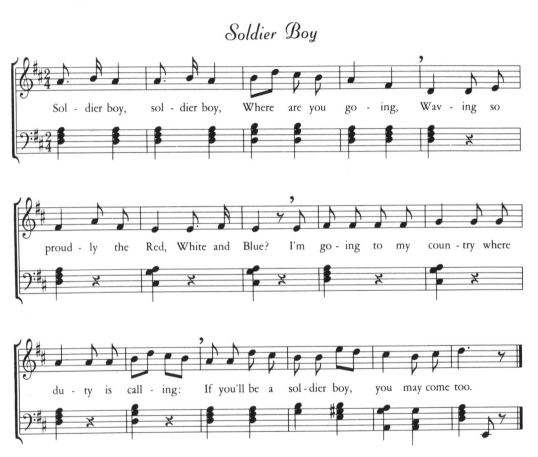

Sol - dier boy, sol - dier boy, Where are you go - ing, Wav - ing so

proud - ly the Red, White and Blue? I'm go - ing to my coun - try where

du - ty is call - ing: If you'll be a sol - dier boy, you may come too.

This action song is especially appropriate for boys. While the class sings the first half of the song, some boy, waving a flag in time to the music, marches around the room. Beginning with the phrase, "I'm going to my country," the boy sings alone and marches until he stands facing another boy to whom he gives the flag as he sings, "you may come, too." The entire action is repeated with the second boy marching and singing and may continue until five or six boys have marched and sung alone.

3

This action provides an excellent means for testing individual rhythmic response as well as individual singing ability, and at the same time preserves the natural, relaxed atmosphere of playing a game.

We'll All Clap Hands Together

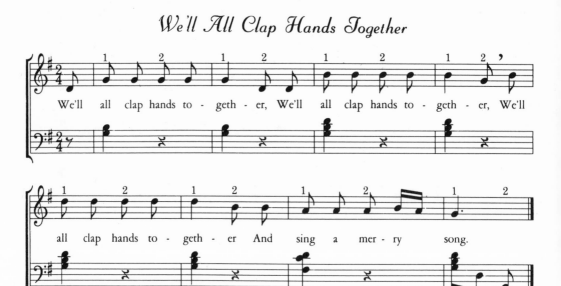

All pupils should stand for this song. Each row or table group selects a leader who is an independent singer. The leaders take their places at the front of the room, each standing directly before his own group.

The leader of the first group sings "We'll all clap hands together" and claps on "1" and "2" as marked in the music. His group sings the second "We'll all clap hands together," clapping on "1" and "2." The entire class finishes the song, clapping on "1" and "2" as they sing.

Without a pause the leader of the next group selects a different movement, such as "We'll all swing arms together," and begins the second stanza. The arms may swing to the left on "1" and to the right on "2." The song is continued with this activity, following the plan for the first stanza.

The leader of the third row continues with another response, such as "We'll all mark time together," stepping lightly in one place with the left foot on "1" and with the right foot on "2". Follow the same plan as with the previous stanzas.

It is important that there be no breaks between these original stanzas. The rhythmic motion should be steady and continuous. Encourage the leaders to invent their own motions in order to keep everyone wondering what the next action will be.

Did You Ever See a Lassie?

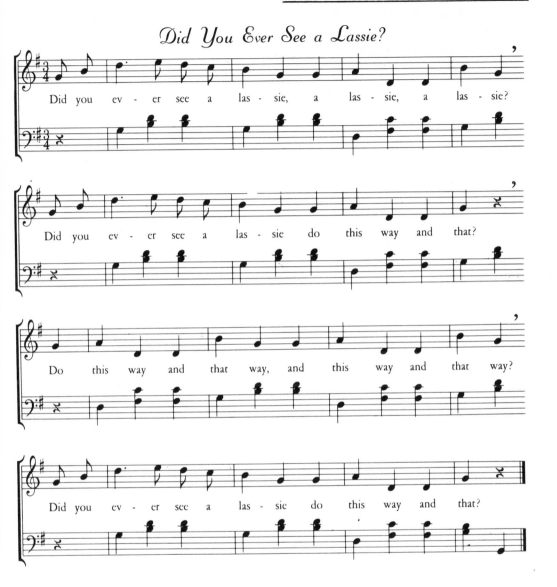

Did you ev-er see a las-sie, a las-sie, a las-sie?

Did you ev-er see a las-sie do this way and that?

Do this way and that way, and this way and that way?

Did you ev-er see a las-sie do this way and that?

This song is especially suitable for girls. The boys, however, sing throughout the song, just as the girls sing with the boys in "Soldier Boy."

One girl is selected as the leader to begin the activity. She decides on some action that will synchronize with the rhythmic swing of the music and demonstrates it as the class sings the first eight measures of the song. During the second half of the song all the children imitate the motions of the leader as they sing, always keeping strictly in time with the music. While the group sings the last four measures of the song, the leader chooses another girl to take her place, and bows

5

or curtsies to her. The entire procedure is repeated, but with a different type of rhythmic movement.

After a few suggestions from the teacher, the girls who act as leaders will begin to demonstrate original ideas in their responses. Some will prefer abstract motions such as swaying the body from side to side with arms extended, or marking time in place on tiptoe, or making a rising and falling motion of the hands. Others will present a rhythmic dramatization of some familiar action, such as rocking the baby, sweeping the floor, or sliding diagonally forward, first with the left foot, then with the right, in imitation of skating.

Bean Porridge Hot

TRADITIONAL MELODY

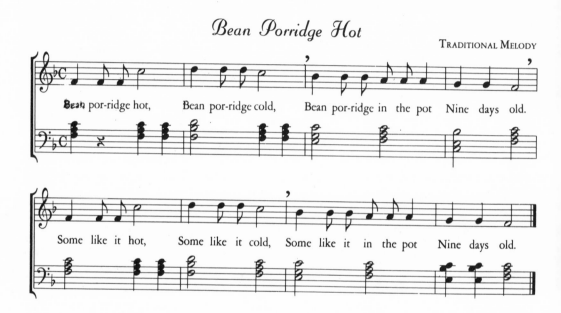

Bean por-ridge hot, Bean por-ridge cold, Bean por-ridge in the pot Nine days old.

Some like it hot, Some like it cold, Some like it in the pot Nine days old.

In this song partners face each other for the rhythmic action, and may either stand or be seated. The movements are synchronized with the words, thus:

"Bean"	- clap hands on thighs;
"porridge"	- clap own hands together;
"hot"	- clap both hands with partner.
"bean porridge cold"	- repeat from the beginning.
"Bean"	- clap hands on thighs;
"porridge"	- clap own hands together;
"in the"	- clap right hand with partner's right;
"pot"	- clap own hands together;
"nine"	- clap left hand with partner's left;
"days"	- clap own hands together;
"old."	- clap both hands with partner.

For the third and fourth phrases, repeat these actions from the beginning.

6

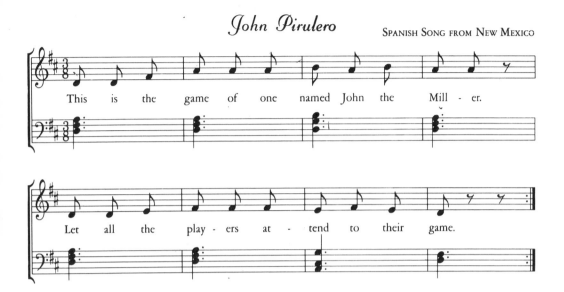

John Pirulero

SPANISH SONG FROM NEW MEXICO

This is the game of one named John the Mill - er.

Let all the play - ers at - tend to their game.

Any number of children can play this game. First choose a leader, who is John the Miller. The others form a circle, sitting cross-legged on the floor. John the Miller sings the song as he stands in the center of the circle. While singing he imitates rhythmically the turning of a millstone. When he finishes he gives each of the others something to do, such as playing a fiddle, washing clothes, sawing wood, and so on. Once in a while John the Miller changes from his grinding to some other action, such as sawing wood. When he does this, the person sawing wood begins grinding the corn. If he does not change his action at once, John the Miller imposes a forfeit, such as hopping on one foot or making a noise like an animal. The game can continue as long as the children want to play.

C. ORIGINAL DRAMATIZATION OF FAMILIAR SONGS

Many teachers can invent rhythmic actions to be used with many other songs, but it is much more desirable to encourage the children to create their own responses. If a song is about a clock, the children may decide to swing their arms as though they were pendulums, or tap "tick" and "tock" with pencils on two different sections of the desk, seat, or table. If the song is about a cobbler, they may pretend they are hammering nails. If the song is about a violin, they may imitate the movements of a violinist, drawing the bow back and forth. It is important that no matter how crude these first creative attempts may be, they should be accepted if they are offered sincerely. Remarkable individual development is

7

frequently the result of successful creative activity of this kind. In all cases, however, the children should be led to sense the need for synchronizing the bodily motion with the rhythmic swing of the music.

Experience with creative rhythmic activity of this kind will lead to an excellent feeling for the dramatization of many songs sung by the children. If the dramatic action is carried out in response to the swing of the music, the result will be highly satisfactory for public performance. With some songs the entire class can enact the dramatization in unison. Other songs, with a story to tell, will be best presented if sung by the class and enacted by a chosen cast. Sometimes the class can form a sort of musical-comedy chorus, doing the singing and a simple rhythmic movement on the refrain, while the cast of characters carries out the dramatic action.

Excellent suggestions for teachers and classes for creative dramatization of songs may be found in Rhythmic Activities, by Annis and Matthews (Ginn and Company), Dramatized Ballads by Tobitt and White (E. P. Dutton and Company), and The Saucy Sailor by Tobitt and White (E. P. Dutton and Company).

The following songs from The World of Music suggest the type of material for starting such creative activity at the various grade levels:

The Friendly Clock	Sing a Song, p. 29
Little Ducky Duddle	Listen and Sing, p. 13
Bouncing Ball	Tuning Up, p. 58
The Woodcutters	Rhythms and Rimes, p. 58
A Queer Business	Songs of Many Lands, p. 27
Drums	Blending Voices, p. 133
The Orchestra	Tunes and Harmonies, p. 183

2. FREE RHYTHMIC ACTIVITY WITH INSTRUMENTAL MUSIC

In one respect physical response to instrumental music is preferable to that which is associated with action songs and singing games. There can be no conflict with tone production. Furthermore, one of the most important phases of rhythmic activity is the development of the child's ability to create his own interpretation of the music he hears. As a means of self-expression and the development of the child's personality, the importance of free creative rhythmic experience can hardly be overestimated.

Rhythms used for free activity by children may be classified as either natural or imitative. Natural rhythms include the familiar movements that are characteristic of children in their everyday experiences, such as walking, running, skipping, and jumping. Imitative rhythms are those imitating the movements of familiar or imaginary beings, animals, or objects in nature, for example, galloping ponies, dancing fairies, mother ironing or sweeping, elephants walking, rabbits hopping, children skating, or trees swaying.

A. PROCEDURE FOR FREE RHYTHMIC ACTIVITY

(1) NATURAL RHYTHM

Several suggestions for making simple responses to music have already been made in connection with action songs. Now the children are asked to listen to music which, without words, suggests certain movements, and then to demonstrate these movements rhythmically.

Many children like to close their eyes while the music is being played, and their response is almost certain to be more original if they do this. When the first selection is played it will probably be wise for the teacher to suggest two or more contrasting movements, one of which quite obviously belongs to the music and can easily be recognized. For example, if she plays music for skipping such as "New-Mown Hay," she may say, "As you listen to this music will you decide whether it tells you to walk slowly or skip?"

Many classes will find it easy to classify the rhythm of this music as they hear it and will be eager to demonstrate what they hear. In this way they have their first experience in the activity of <u>listening</u> to the music in order to discover what it suggests. No such experience occurs if the teacher simply tells the class that she is about to play some music for skipping. Every possible opportunity should be given for the children to listen independently and then interpret the music for themselves. Only in this way will they develop any of the power of close attention to music that is so essential if they are to respond rhythmically.

(Play a Tune, p. 10)

New-Mown Hay

ENGLISH FOLK TUNE

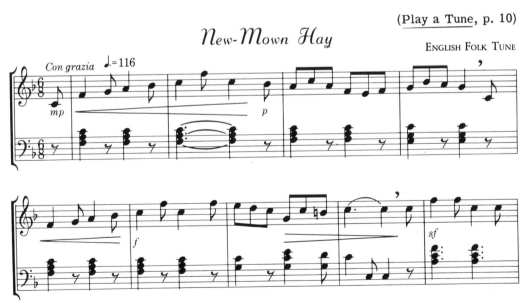

9

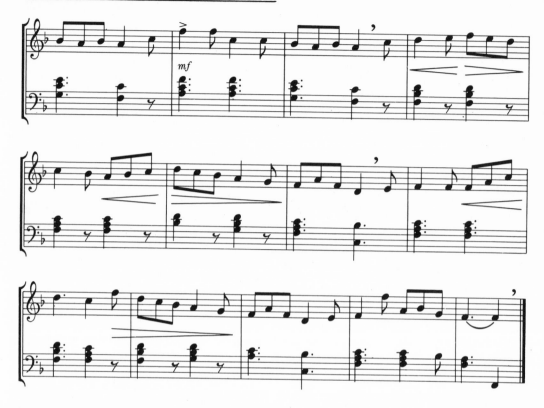

As soon as any child definitely feels the movement of skipping while the music is being played, he should demonstrate the motion as the music continues. This may be done in the aisles or in a circle, according to the arrangement of the room.

The next piece to be played should be a contrasting rhythm, such as "La Cinquantaine" (walk), or "Dance of the Moorish Slaves" (run). (See page 26.) Other selections suitable for these activities appear on pages in Chapters II and III.

La Cinquantaine

GABRIEL-MARIE

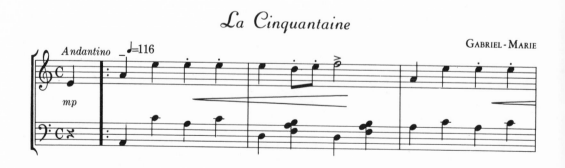

10

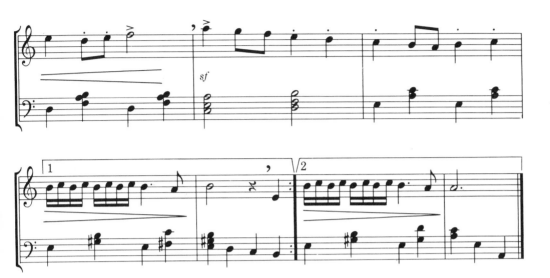

Before long the class will be able to distinguish many familiar rhythms such as skipping, galloping, running, marching, and walking at different rates of speed, and will enjoy demonstrating them. Where younger children are concerned, skips, gallops, and runs are usually the most natural rhythms for the first experiences. The children should form the habit of listening to a few measures of each selection before attempting any physical response. Much of the disorder that sometimes accompanies this type of activity can be avoided if a definite routine is established for listening and responding to each musical selection. These suggestions for a possible routine are given.

Children who are to respond to the music with bodily movement are standing. Other members of the class are seated, prepared to keep time to the music by some simple, small movement.

Teacher: "Ready. Listen!"

Pupils standing and those in their seats close eyes and listen.

Teacher plays enough of the music to establish the rhythm definitely. Probably eight measures will be sufficient. Then without stopping the music she gives the direction, "Move." Children open their eyes and start moving in time with the music, those standing responding with free bodily motions, and those in their seats quietly where they are.

In the early experiences or when a new and complicated idea is presented, it is frequently best to stop for a brief discussion before giving the direction to move. After the discussion the routine can be continued, "Listen! Move."

Older pupils, even when this type of activity is unfamiliar to them, frequently enjoy demonstrating the movements suggested by the music as much as the little children. In cases of shyness pupils may prefer to remain seated and show the ideas suggested by the music with free motions of arms and hands. Sometimes the use of rhythm instruments will arouse the interest of older children and give them the necessary fundamental experience with movement and lead them to try other free bodily movements.

(2) IMITATIVE RHYTHM

Imitative rhythms are very popular, especially with small children. Some children may be confused by the idea that music may indicate some motions such as walking or galloping. But when the rhythm of an elephant's walk is compared with that of a galloping pony the idea becomes clear and concrete. One composition may suggest an elephant, in which case the child may walk slowly and rhythmically with head bent forward and the arms (palms of hands together) swinging slowly in time to the music in imitation of an elephant's trunk.

Another selection may suggest trees swaying in the wind. The children may hold their arms high as though they were branches and sway with the rhythmic swing of the music. Still another composition may arouse a desire to dance on tiptoe as fairies do. If an instrumental selection is being played on the phonograph, the pupils may pretend to play the violin, trombone, or drum with the music, or they may be band leaders, keeping time with arm movements. Another valuable and popular type of rhythmic response is the imitation of the see-saw or mill wheel, done by standing and raising the arms so that they are on a level with the shoulders and then moving with the music.

The child's freedom of interpretation should be considered constantly during all of this activity. Some particular selection may suggest a lullaby, both to the composer and the teacher, but it may make one child think of a tall tree swaying back and forth in the breeze, while another may imagine that it is "see-saw" music. If the interpretations of individuals are accepted and the members of the class are asked to choose the rhythmic movement which they feel best expresses the music, a sense of musical discrimination is established. This will continue to grow as experience increases. The variety of responses is limited only by the music available (phonograph records or piano music), the pianistic ability and resourcefulness of the teacher, and the imagination of the pupils.

B. PROVISION FOR INDIVIDUAL DIFFERENCES

If a child has difficulty in keeping time to the music he should receive special attention and have a great deal of rhythmic experience. The teacher should remember that each child has his own natural rhythm, and should watch the group movements to make sure that the tempo of the music is suitable for the majority of those who are participating. The large proportion of children will respond smoothly if the music is played in a tempo which is natural for them and if the rhythmic movement is familiar to them.

An individual who does not move in time to the music should not be classified as lacking in a sense of rhythm. His rhythmic sense may be good but he may not have discovered that the pulsations in the music he is hearing move at a different speed from that which characterizes his usual movements. Frequently he will begin to sense the rhythm if the tempo at which the music is being played is retarded or accelerated to fit his personal speed of movement. For example, if a child cannot walk with the music of "La Cinquantaine," the teacher should watch him and play slower or faster in order that the music may follow his steps. After a good deal of experience of this kind, when the child has clearly sensed this feeling of synchronizing his movements with the rhythmic swing of the music, the speed of the playing can be changed to the faster or slower tempo suitable for the rest of the class and he will gradually learn to adjust his movements both to the rhythm and the tempo of the music heard. Marching with other children who keep in step with the music may also help the child who is not accurate in his responses.

C. A MUSICAL GAME, "FOLLOW THE LEADER"

Groups of all ages will enjoy and will gain valuable rhythmic experience from participating in a musical game of "Follow the Leader." The music used should have strong, steady rhythmic pulsations. The leader stands before the class and starts making a simple rhythmic movement in time to the music. The class follows him, using the same movement. Frequently and without warning, the leader changes to a different type of rhythmic motion, the class always imitating him. It is possible to conduct this activity with the group seated, or standing in place, or it is possible to have them follow the leader around the room if greater freedom is desired.

A few minutes of this musical "Follow the Leader" can provide a great deal of refreshing, relaxing activity for a class, even when the pupils remain in their seats. Perhaps the leader will start by marking time lightly, suddenly change to a body sway with hands overhead, then change again, this time shaking the right hand lightly, always following the rhythmic swing of the music.

D. MUSIC FOR FREE RHYTHMIC ACTIVITY

For some rhythmic activities suggested in later chapters, the choice of music to be sung or played is limited to that which uses only certain measures or note

13

values. There are no such limitations, however, placed on the music to be used for the activities described in this section. Music in many different kinds of measures and with various kinds of note values may be used, as long as it has a smooth, even flow of rhythmic pulsations. In addition to the music included in this chapter, much of that found in later chapters, especially Chapters II and III, is suitable for free rhythmic activity. Many other suitable selections also are to be found in the collection Play a Tune from the World of Music Series. Some of these are listed herewith:

Skips and Gallops

Gigue	Corelli	p. 7
Queen of the Peris	Aubert	p. 8
Hunting Song	Schumann	p. 9
I'll Tend My Sheep	French Folk Tune	p. 10
Dancing Sunbeams	Leavitt	p. 12
Bagatelle No. 5	Beethoven	p. 16
Sicilienne, Opus 68, No. 11	Schumann	p. 15
Siciliana from Violin Sonata	Weber	p. 13

Runs

Song of the Shepherdess	Weber	p. 20
Scherzo, Opus 16, No. 2	Mendelssohn	p. 21
Rondo, Viennese Sonata	Mozart	p. 22
La Roxelane	Haydn	p. 23
Momento Capriccioso	Weber	p. 24

Walks

Folk Dance	Danish Folk Tune	p. 25
Jack Be Nimble	Strickland	p. 69
Gavotte	Gossec	p. 26
Musette	Gluck	p. 28
Seventeenth-Century Dance	English Folk Tune	p. 66
Minuet for Harpischord	Purcell	p. 26
Minuet	Scharwenka	p. 28
Moslem Swords	Strickland	p. 73

Marches

March from The Queen of Sheba	Gounod	p. 31
March from Leonore	Raff	p. 32
Forward March	Italian Folk Tune	p. 33
Cavalry March	Finnish Folk Tune	p. 36
Christmas Tree March	Gade	p. 35
Norwegian Dance	Grieg	p. 39
Ecossaise No. 3	Schubert	p. 30
Rondo from Sextette, Opus 71	Beethoven	p. 30

In general, much of the music to be used for imitative rhythms can be chosen from the same lists as are used for natural rhythms. Thus the music for a slow walk may well be interpreted as an elephant's walk; that for running may become an elves' dance; while what is sometimes used for swaying, or skipping, or galloping, may, with a little imagination, be made to fit any number of possible dramatic situations. |All of the music used should be played with a definite accent, so that the pupils can sense the swing and the pulsations without difficulty. At the same time, care should be exercised not to overemphasize the accent so that the music becomes mechanical.

If the teacher wishes to use phonograph records, many of the selections listed are available in this form. An examination of the record catalogs of different companies or a letter to the educational department of one of the companies will provide a list of recordings (either single titles or record sets) which may be used effectively for the rhythmic activities suggested here.

3. RHYTHM INSTRUMENTS

The playing of rhythm instruments by children at different grade levels, older as well as younger, can be one of the most important and popular factors in rhythmic development. It should be kept in mind that the activities suggested here, whether for rhythm band or for special rhythm instruments, are planned as an integral, contributing part of the school music program, and not as a separate project designed to provide performing groups on programs.

Discussions in this chapter are concerned only with the use of rhythm instruments in the development of the children's power to make simple response to musical rhythms. Later chapters include rhythm-instrument activities of a greater variety and degree of difficulty.

A. THE RHYTHM BAND

The rhythm band is one of the most enjoyable of rhythmic activities, and has real educational value when it is made a project that is both rhythmic and creative. The experience it provides justifies not only the financial expenditure that may be necessary for the instruments, but also a definite time in the school program to provide time for the activity.

Many teachers have found that it is advantageous to have the rhythm-band period scheduled immediately following recess or the opening of school, so that the instruments can be in place on desks or tables when the children enter the room. Then if a march is played at the close of the period, each child can put his own instrument away, playing it until he reaches the shelf or box where it belongs, and returning quietly to his seat.

As in the teaching of action songs and folk games, the aim of the rhythm band is to develop the children's feeling for the rhythmic swing of the music and their

15

LEARNING MUSIC THROUGH RHYTHM

ability to make muscular response to it. As with these other activities, it may require some time to accomplish this with all children, but if it is not accomplished the time and effort spent on the rhythm band will have been wasted in so far as musical results or educational benefits are concerned. If the group seems slow in learning to use the instruments rhythmically, it may be that the teacher has attempted to push them too fast, or to use activities that are too complicated for beginners.

These first rhythm-band lessons will be spent only in giving the children opportunity to learn how to handle the instruments and to play them in time to the music. It will be wise to ask the class to accompany the music softly. This admonition is especially important with those instruments which can be noisy if carelessly handled. Individual help will frequently be needed in the handling of instruments that require special muscular skill. At successive rehearsals of the rhythm band, children should be given different instruments to play in order that they may become accustomed to handling all of them. No child enjoys playing the same instrument constantly, and each instrument requires a certain type of movement and therefore gives a special type of training in muscular co-ordination. Later, when a definite orchestration is worked out for a selection, each child will learn to take his place, playing a certain instrument whenever this particular music is used. In this beginning period, however, the class simply listens to the music and tries to play an instrument in response to the rhythm of the music. Therefore a frequent change of instruments is important.

Any music (piano or phonograph) that has a good rhythmic swing is usable for these first lessons on the rhythm band. The selections included in this and other chapters of this book will be found suitable for this activity. The foundation work in rhythm band can also be carried on with rhythmic songs. However, the songs must, as was suggested in the case of action songs, be thoroughly familiar before they are used for such an activity.

When the children have acquired considerable skill in playing the instruments in time to a variety of rhythms, usually they automatically become conscious of obvious loud and soft sections in the music, or of verse and chorus sections in songs. They will soon learn to divide their instruments roughly into two groups (perhaps loud and soft) and plan the orchestration of the music with this in mind. Some children may begin to pick out the little rhythm patterns they hear in the music, but in general all of this work is done with no attempt at any response except to the smooth, rhythmic swing of the music. Further experience will lead to a greater variety of activities, which are discussed in the following chapters.

B. SPECIAL RHYTHM INSTRUMENTS

Aside from the traditional rhythm band, the use of special rhythm instruments, sometimes singly, sometimes in groups, has great importance in the fundamental rhythm experience of any class. Even where a good set of rhythm band instruments is available, the children will enjoy choosing just one instrument which seems especially suitable for a song or instrumental selection. With this instrument they can accompany the free rhythmic activities described earlier in this chapter.

Older boys and girls may have little interest in the rhythm band as an organization, but they will take great pleasure in learning to play a few distinctive instruments which suit the mood or nationality of the songs they are singing or the dances they are learning. Many a sixth-grader who was too tense to be able to follow the music in simple marching or dancing has finally had his rhythmic sense awakened through the experience of being one of several who played a simple rhythmic accompaniment to the music for a song or dance that was Latin American, Indian, or perhaps Chinese in origin or in mood. There is no instrument quite like a hand drum or tom tom for inspiring children to follow the swing of the music to which they are singing or listening. Many boys learn to keep time to music for the first time as they play instruments they have constructed for themselves--whether crude Indian rattles, or beautifully constructed jungle drums.

As a combination of creative activity and simple, fundamental rhythmic movement, this work with special rhythm instruments can be one of the most valuable of the rhythmic activities. It flourishes in proportion to the imagination and ingenuity of both teacher and class.

4. FOLK DANCES AND GAMES

A. PROCEDURES FOR TRADITIONAL GAMES

Children of all ages enjoy folk dances and games. Some of the simpler ones can be presented very early as a means of increasing the experience in feeling the rhythmic swing of the music. The following are included here as typical examples of easy folk games which emphasize a full, free bodily movement in time to the music:

Shoemaker's Dance
Chimes of Dunkirk
Dance of Greeting
I See You
Skip to My Lou
Four in a Boat

17

Shoemaker's Dance

DANISH

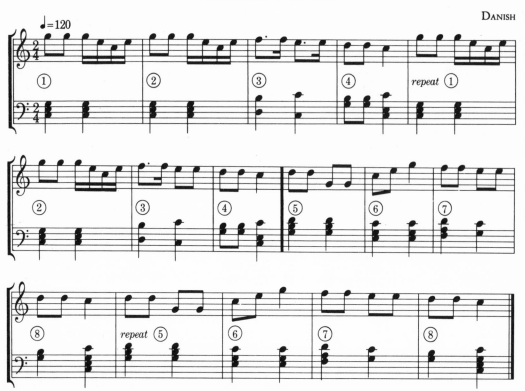

Partners form a double circle and face each other.

Measure 1: <u>Wind thread</u> - With elbows high, hold clenched fists in front of the chest and revolve them around each other rapidly.

Measure 2: <u>Reverse</u> - Without pausing, reverse the movement.

Measure 3: <u>Wax thread</u> - Jerk the elbows back twice during the measure, each time also lifting the left knee and saying "So, so."

Measure 4: <u>Pegging</u> - Strike left fist with the right fist three times, saying "Rap, rap, rap."

Measures 1-4 are repeated with movements as above.

Measures 5-8: <u>Skip</u> - Partners join inside hands and skip around the circle counterclockwise, outside hands on hips.

Turn around and repeat measure 5-8, skipping clockwise.

Repeat the entire action from the beginning.

Chimes of Dunkirk

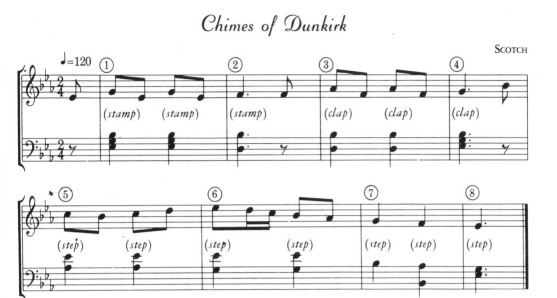

Partners form a double circle, facing each other, with hands on hips.

Measures 1 and 2: Stamp three times.

Measures 3 and 4: Clap hands three times.

Measures 5 and 6: Partners join hands, take four slow running steps in place (one to each beat), beginning with the left foot.

Measures 7 and 8: Partners release hands; each dancer takes three slow running steps (one to each beat) to the left, and faces a new partner.

Repeat from the beginning.

Dance of Greeting

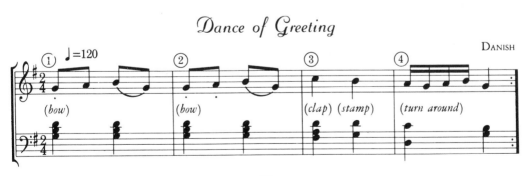

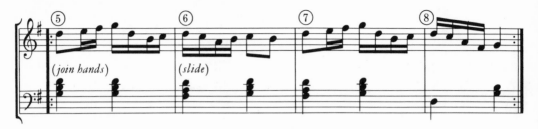

A circle is formed with partners standing, all facing center.

Measure 1: Bow to partner.

Measure 2: Bow to neighbor.

Measure 3: Clap on the first beat and stamp on the second beat.

Measure 4: Turn around.

Repeat measures 1-4.

Measures 5-8: All join hands and face left. All slide to the left, starting with the left foot.

Repeat measures 5-8 without pausing and with hands still joined, facing right and all sliding right, starting with the right foot.

I See You

SWEDISH

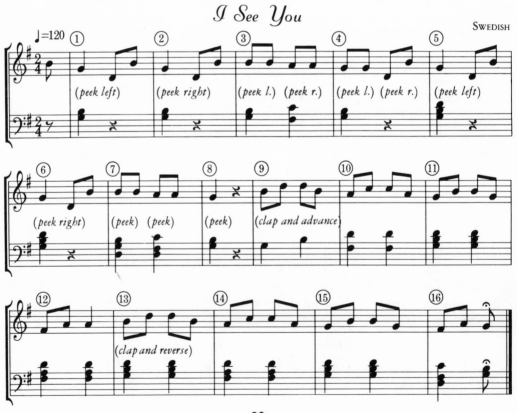

20

Dancers form two double lines, six to eight feet apart.

      B - Boy   G - Girl

Back row: B B B B
Front row: G G G G

Front row: B B B B
Back row: G G G G

These double lines face each other. The children in the front row place hands on hips. Those in the back row place hands on the shoulders of children in front of them.

Measure 1: Children in the back row move heads to left, peeking over the shoulders of those in front at the dancers opposite them, who are doing the same thing.

Measure 2: Reverse the action for measure 1, peeking over the right shoulders.

Measures 3-4: Back rows peek four times instead of twice, alternately over left and right shoulders (left and right in measure 3; left and right in measure 4).

Measures 5-8: Repeat actions for measures 1-4.

Measures 9-10: Children in the back row remove hands from shoulders of those in front, clap once on the first beat, then move quickly forward at left of partner into the open space, and grasp right hands or link elbows of right arms of children who are advancing at the same time from the opposite back row.

Measures 11-12: The couples dance to the left, clockwise, around.

Measures 14-16: Dance in the opposite direction. On the hold in the 16th measure, the children return to their original positions, except that those who were in the back row take their places in the front row, and vice versa.

Repeat the entire dance in the new positions.

This dance may be made a singing game by using the following words:

> I see you, I see you,
> Tra la, la, la, la, la, la, la,
> I see you, I see you,
> Tra la, la, la, la, la.
>
> You see me, and I see you,
> Then you take me, and I'll take you,
> You see me, and I see you,
> Then you take me, and I'll take you.

(On Wings of Song, p. 82)

Four in a Boat

TRADITIONAL SINGING GAME

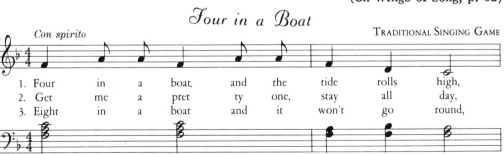

1. Four in a boat, and the tide rolls high,
2. Get me a pretty one, stay all day,
3. Eight in a boat and it won't go round,

21

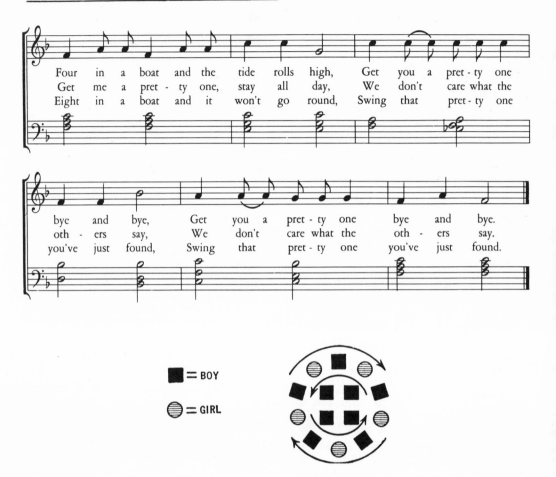

Four in a boat and the tide rolls high, Get you a pret-ty one
Get me a pret-ty one, stay all day, We don't care what the
Eight in a boat and it won't go round, Swing that pret-ty one

bye and bye, Get you a pret-ty one bye and bye.
oth - ers say, We don't care what the oth - ers say.
you've just found, Swing that pret-ty one you've just found.

■ = BOY

⊜ = GIRL

Formation: Outer circle--hands joined, facing center. Inner circle--four boys, hands joined, facing outer circle.

Action (Verse 1): Outer circle walks to the left (clockwise). Inner circle walks to the right (counterclockwise).

Action (Verse 2): All drop hands and both circles walk to the left (clockwise). Each boy in the center chooses from the outside circle the girl who is nearest him and walks beside her until the end of the verse.

Action (Verse 3): Each boy in the center pulls his partner into the inner circle. Members of both circles join hands and walk in opposite directions as in the first verse. Players pantomime action "Eight in a boat and it won't go round" until the last line, when all boys swing their partners once around. Then each boy in the inner circle leaves his partner and retires to the outer circle. Repeat the entire song with girls in the center.

Skip to My Lou

(On Wings of Song, p. 11)

TRADITIONAL SINGING GAME

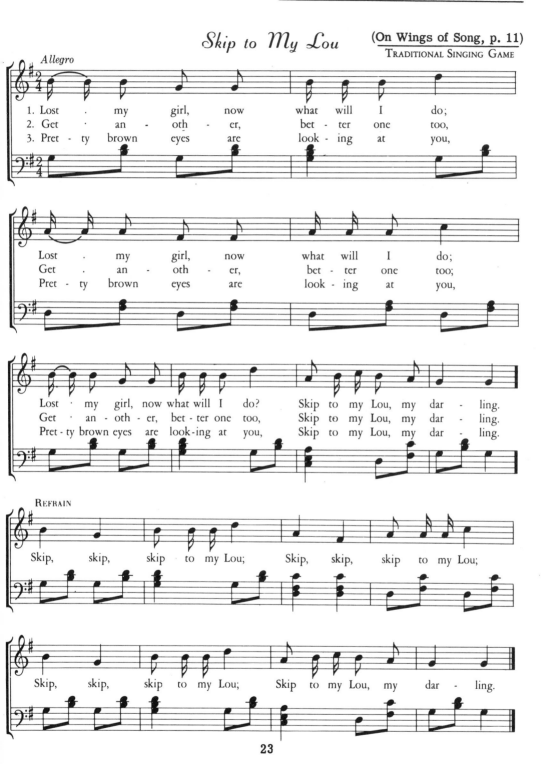

1. Lost my girl, now what will I do;
2. Get an-oth-er, bet-ter one too,
3. Pret-ty brown eyes are look-ing at you,

Lost my girl, now what will I do;
Get an-oth-er, bet-ter one too;
Pret-ty brown eyes are look-ing at you,

Lost my girl, now what will I do? Skip to my Lou, my dar-ling.
Get an-oth-er, bet-ter one too, Skip to my Lou, my dar-ling.
Pret-ty brown eyes are look-ing at you, Skip to my Lou, my dar-ling.

REFRAIN

Skip, skip, skip to my Lou; Skip, skip, skip to my Lou;

Skip, skip, skip to my Lou; Skip to my Lou, my dar-ling.

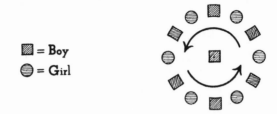

■ = Boy

◉ = Girl

Formation: Single circle of partners, facing the center. The girl is at her partner's right. An extra boy, without a partner, is inside the circle.

Action: All sing and clap hands while the boy in the center chooses someone's partner. They take skating position with right hands joined, crossed over with joined left hands and skip to the right (counterclockwise) around the circle until the first verse and chorus are completed. Then they return to vacated places in the circle. Just before the chorus is ended, the boy without a partner chooses a girl and repeats the action during the second verse and chorus. This continues for the entire song.

B. CREATIVE ACTIVITY IN FOLK-DANCE STYLE

The folk dance and singing game offer another opportunity for encouraging and developing the pupils' creative power. After the pupils have learned two or three dances (as taught by the teacher), they will be interested to try inventing original steps and phrase activities. Sometimes these will be new steps to familiar dance tunes; again they may be original dance arrangements to music for which there are no traditional dance steps. While the first results may lack some of the clearcut form and smooth organization of the usual folk dance, these original creations are very valuable because they are the expressions of the pupils themselves. Intent listening and careful thinking are necessary if the music is to make a vivid impression on the child. Ability in self-expression and the capacity to listen with discrimination will grow in proportion to the opportunities which the teacher provides for individual creative effort.

Through all these creative experiences, the teacher should act as a sympathetic member of the group, helping and guiding the child's efforts so that the result may be constructive and satisfying.

Chapter II
Responses to the Natural Rhythms
in Music Heard

The distinction between natural and imitative rhythms has already been explained (pp. 8-12). It is expected that the activities outlined in this chapter will have been preceded by a great variety of rhythmic experiences with games, dances, free rhythmic expression, and the use of rhythm instruments as suggested in Chapter I. Before this new type of activity is begun the majority of the pupils in the class should be able to respond accurately to the rhythmic pulsations in the music with simple movements such as are included in the activities described in Chapter I.

1. THREE FUNDAMENTAL RHYTHMS

Only the natural rhythms of walking, running, and skipping are used for the activities presented in this chapter. The purpose of these activities is to make the children conscious of the notes in the music to which they are listening. Their previous experience has been concerned with responses to the general rhythmic flow of the music. Now they begin to give close attention to the different kinds of notes that make the rhythmic pattern. Because of this fact the choice of music for this work is most important.

A. PROCEDURE

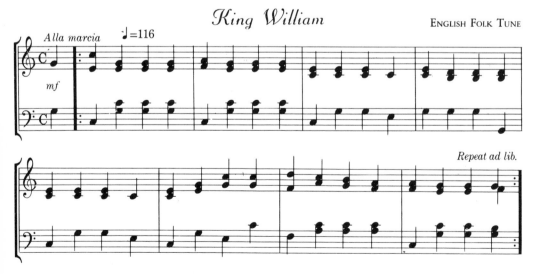

King William

ENGLISH FOLK TUNE

Alla marcia ♩=116

mf

Repeat ad lib.

25

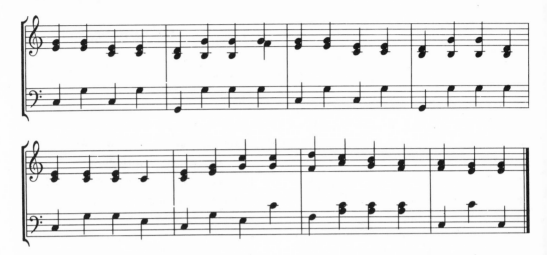

(1) RESPONSE ON THE FLOOR

The teacher plays "King William" on the piano and the children listen to decide what familiar movement the music suggests. It is probable that after their previous experience they will immediately recognize that the rhythm of the music suggests walking. As they respond by walking they may discover that it is possible to make their feet do just what the notes in the music are doing.

A contrasting rhythm such as "Dance of the Moorish Slaves" follows immediately, for recognition and response. Emphasis should be placed on listening for the running movement suggested by the notes as they are heard in the music.

Dance of the Moorish Slaves (Play a Tune, p. 20)

GIUSEPPE VERDI

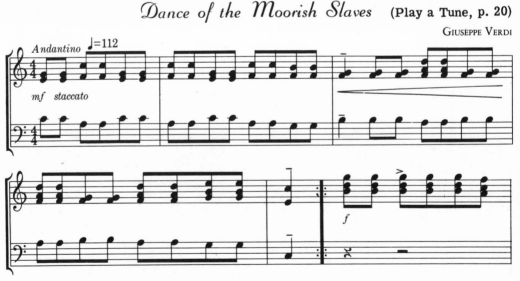

26

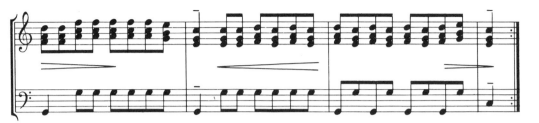

Follow this at once with a skipping rhythm such as

Turkey in the Straw

TRADITIONAL

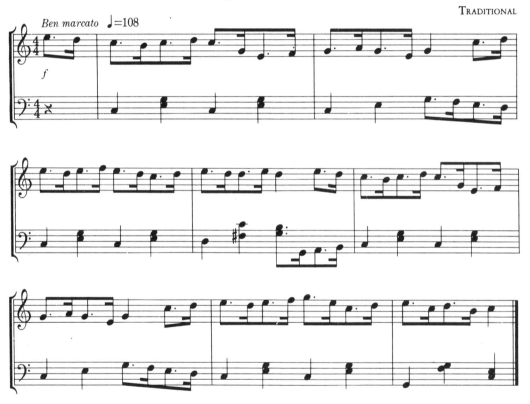

There is little that is actually new in the activities of this chapter except a concentration on the three fundamental rhythms of walking, running, and skipping as a preparation for music reading, and a gradually increasing emphasis on attention to the notes heard as the music is played, as well as to the general rhythmic flow of the music. The importance of these activities cannot be overestimated; they are essential to success with more advanced activities which come later.

LEARNING MUSIC THROUGH RHYTHM

At this stage of development only one natural rhythm at a time should be used. The music should come to a complete stop between the different rhythms, and should not yet proceed directly from walking to skipping or running. This will assure the development of a habit of listening to the music before making any response.

(2) RESPONSE AT SEATS

It is sometimes impossible or undesirable to have the entire class on the floor at the same time. The teacher may be able to give attention to an individual or a small group better than to the whole class. Some form of rhythmic response should be suggested to the children who remain in their places. Sometimes they may "walk," "run," or "skip" with their arms and hands while they remain seated. The walking rhythm will usually be a free down-swing of the forearm: "down, down, walk, walk," and so on, the entire arm from the shoulder taking part in the movement. The skipping and running rhythms, being faster, will be smaller movements, using more of hand and wrist motion.

Frequently these children prefer to walk, run, or skip in place beside their chairs, or in the aisle beside their seats. Perhaps they themselves can invent some other satisfactory method of showing, at their seats, that they feel the movement suggested by the music.

B. CHOICE OF MUSIC FOR NATURAL RHYTHMS

The selections included in this chapter have been chosen to meet the requirements listed below. Additional material for similar use is to be found in Chapter III.

(1) WALKING

It is strongly recommended that the music used for the walking activities in this chapter include only selections in 2/4, 3/4, or 4/4 measure, in which the melody (played by the right hand) consists almost entirely of quarter notes. Some musical examples, in addition to "King William", on page 25, follows:

German Dance

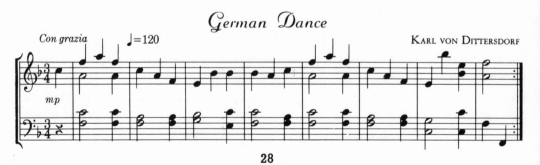

Con grazia ♩ ♩ ♩=120   KARL VON DITTERSDORF

mp

28

Lady Fair

FRENCH FOLK TUNE

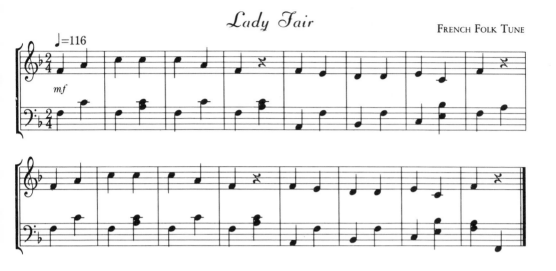

Also these selections in Chapter III are suitable:

Folk Melody, p. 37
Hungarian Folk Tune, p. 43
Russian Hymn, p. 47

(2) RUNNING

Music for this experience should be confined to 2/4, 3/4, or 4/4 measure in which the melody consists almost entirely of eighth notes. Examples are "Dance of the Moorish Slaves," p. 26, and the following:

Scherzino

MORITZ MOSZKOWSKI

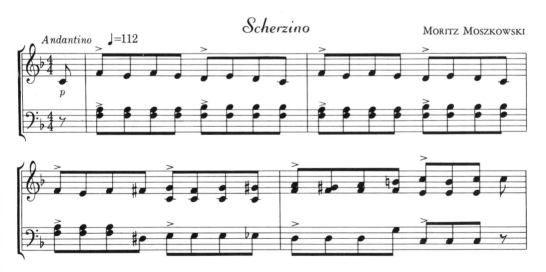

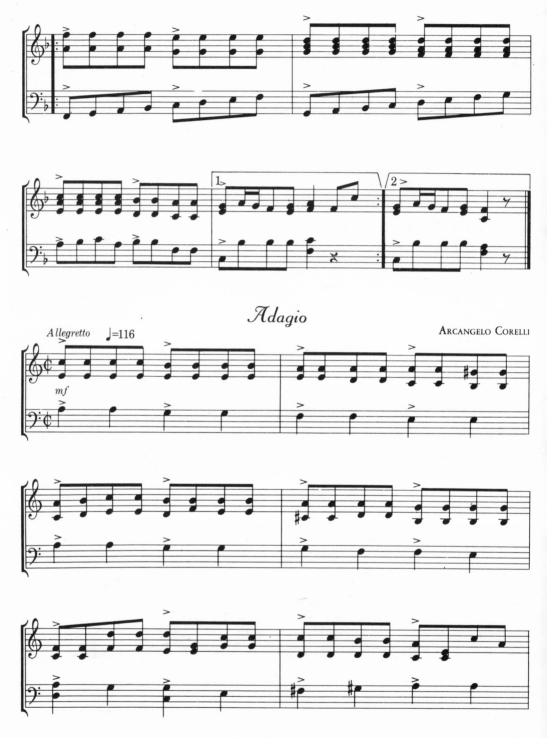

Adagio

ARCANGELO CORELLI

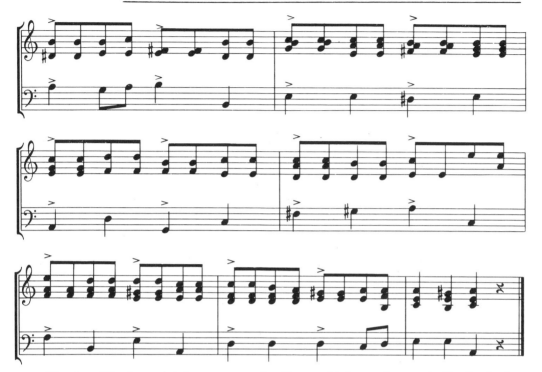

Chapter III also contains some selections which can be used effectively for running. They are found under the following titles:

(3) SKIPPING

Music used for skipping usually has one of the following beat groups or patterns predominating in the right-hand melody line:

a. ♩. ♪ in 2/4, 3/4, and 4/4 measure:

Old Country Dance

AMERICAN TRADITIONAL

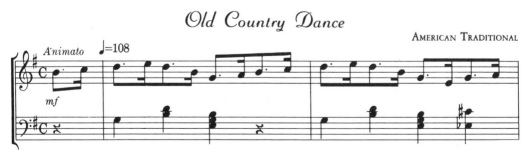

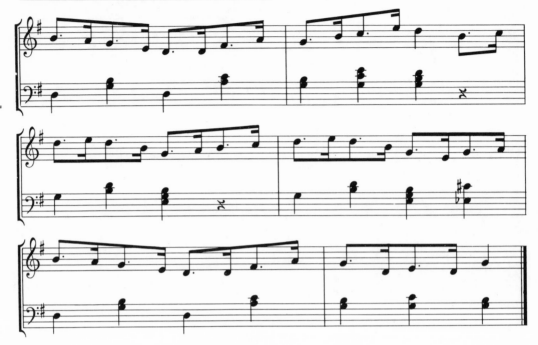

b. ♩ ♪ or ♩♪ in fast 6/8, 9/8, or 12/8 measure:

Wooden Shoes

FRENCH FOLK TUNE

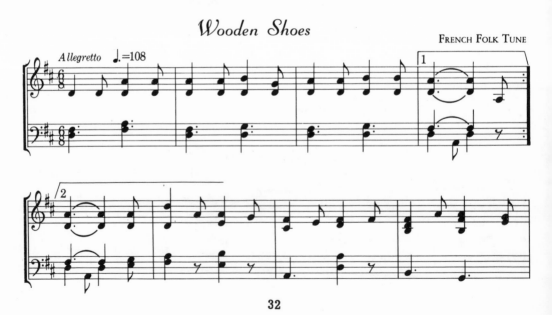

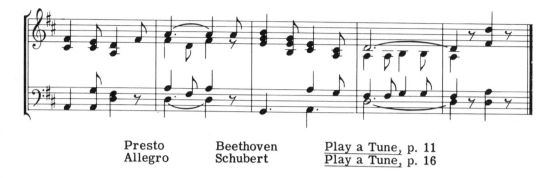

| Presto | Beethoven | Play a Tune, p. 11 |
| Allegro | Schubert | Play a Tune, p. 16 |

C. ADAPTING MUSIC TO DIFFERENT RHYTHMS

It will be a distinct advantage if the teacher is able to improvise or adapt music or rhythmic patterns for these activities instead of playing the same selections over and over again. If a certain melody is used always in the same way, some children will identify it as one of the "walking" or one of the "skipping" tunes. This is easily prevented if the teacher uses some of these selections or some from other chapters which are suitable, playing them not only as written for walking, but also for skipping or running.

The suggestions which follow are made for the help of the teacher who has had little keyboard experience. Here is a simple selection for walking:

Theme

MOZART

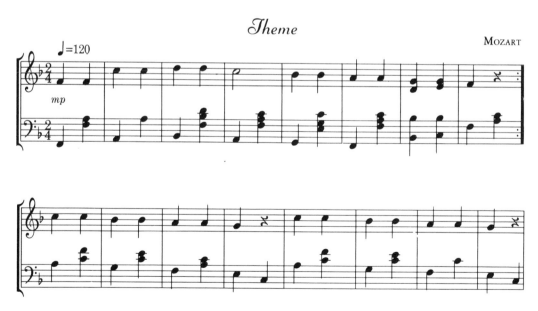

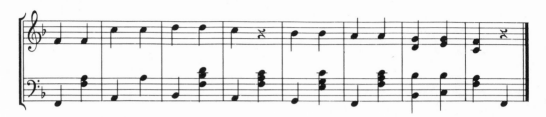

It is possible to adjust this simple walking theme so that it is appropriate for skipping by substituting the rhythmic pattern ♪. ♪ for each quarter note, thus:

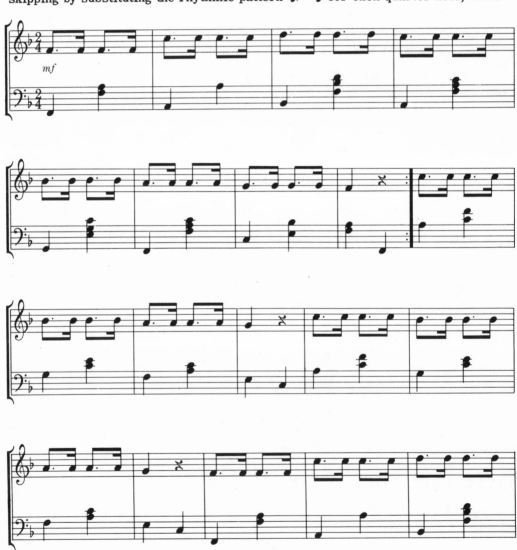

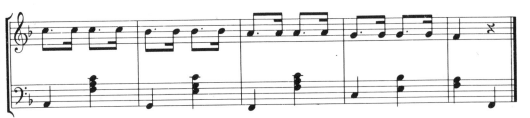

Another change or adjustment is to substitute 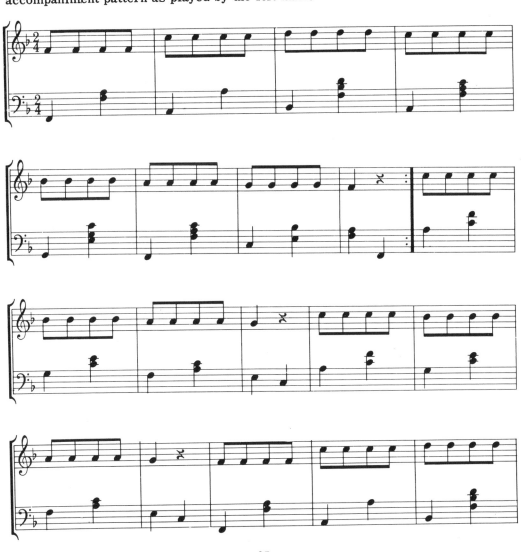 for each quarter note, thus making the music appropriate for running. No change should be made in the accompaniment pattern as played by the left hand.

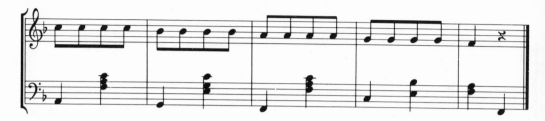

D. USE OF RHYTHM INSTRUMENTS

To give variety it is sometimes desirable to use a rhythm instrument instead of the piano. A good hand drum or tom-tom with clear, deep tone will usually be the most satisfactory choice for these earliest experiences. The teacher can easily sound a series of walking, skipping, or running tones on the drum, while the children respond through movement. The rhythmic patterns already suggested, as well as the selections given in this chapter, can be used.

All children will enjoy playing these on a drum if one is available for their use, but only those whose rhythmic sense and muscular co-ordination allow them to produce a steady, evenly pulsating pattern should play for the class to follow in rhythmic response. If pupils are asked to respond to poor, erratic rhythmic patterns the result will be confusion on the part of the children who have not yet developed good power of rhythmic response, and inattention and disciplinary troubles from the class in general.

E. RHYTHMIC NOTATION

Some teachers prefer to introduce the notation of these rhythmic groups concurrently with the children's response to them. While satisfactory results may sometimes be accomplished by so doing, it is recommended that much experience in physical movement precede the presentation of the notation, in accordance with the principle of the thing before the sign. Therefore the presentation of these rhythms with their notation is not introduced until Chapter VIII.

Chapter III
Changing from One Natural Rhythm
to Another

As soon as the children are able to distinguish easily between the natural rhythms suggested by the music they hear, and are able to show this by rhythmic response, they are ready to proceed to the use of music in which the rhythms change without warning.

A. PROCEDURE

(1) RESPONSE ON THE FLOOR

The children who are to participate on the floor stand in a line or in a circle, ready for the music to start. No warning is given that there is to be anything new or different about the music to be heard. The teacher simply plays the series of three different rhythms which follow this paragraph without stopping, going from one to another without the slightest break or hesitation, and the children start to respond as usual, first listening, then moving.

Folk Melody

GERMAN

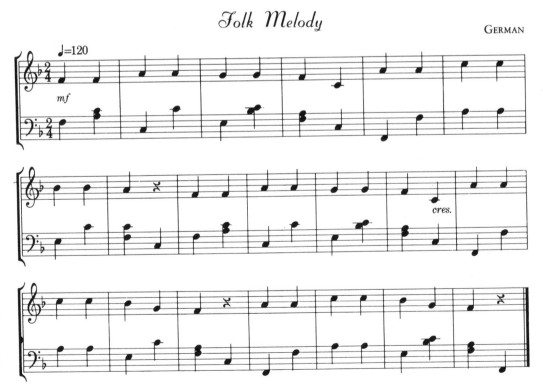

Etude

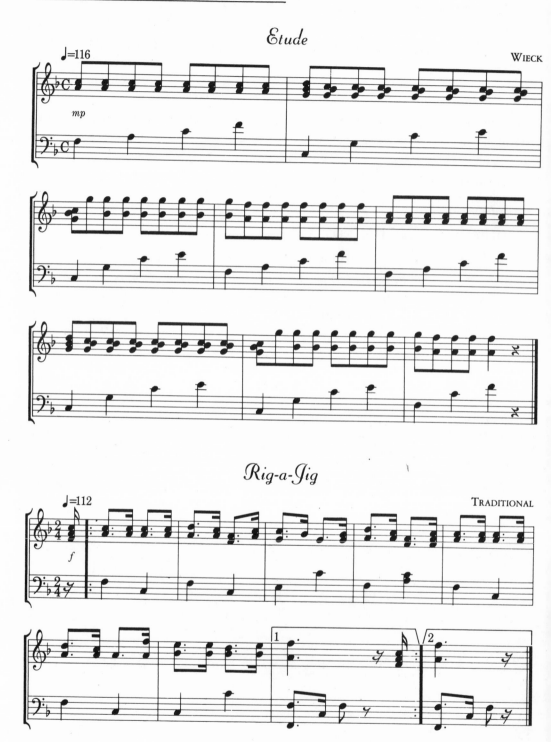

In case none of the children detect these changes in rhythm, it is best to stop the music entirely. The stopping of the music should be the signal always for an immediate cessation of all activity - complete quiet in the room. Then, if the children stand quietly and listen to the music as it moves from one rhythm to another, they will usually recognize the changes as they take place. Sometimes it is helpful to suggest that all close their eyes as they listen, just as they did in the first experience with free rhythmic activity (p. 9). After standing in place and listening quietly to the music there will seldom be any further difficulty in responding accurately as the rhythmic changes occur.

It should not be necessary for the teacher to call attention to these changing rhythms in the music. If the rhythms are played, either on piano or drum, with clear, well-defined accents, and some children still cannot discover the changes independently, they have not had enough previous experience with separate rhythms as outlined in Chapter II.

In changing from one rhythm to another it is essential that the transition be smooth and that not a beat be lost. Otherwise the break in the music may reveal the change in the rhythm. Children soon grasp the idea that the music may change in rhythmic suggestion at any time, and that they must always listen carefully and attentively while responding to it by walking, skipping or running in order to change the response when necessary. This is an important step in their development because it will serve as the foundation for ability which will be needed later when they are asked to give close attention to the music in the study of measure and note values.

(2) RESPONSE AT SEATS

As was suggested on page 28, it is sometimes impossible or undesirable for every pupil in the room actually to walk, skip or run to the music. However, there should always be some form of response for those who remain seated, in order that each child may participate constantly in every activity. Several possible responses for those who remain in their places have been suggested on pages 28 - 33 in Chapter II. The same concentration is required if the children who remain seated are to follow the changing rhythms with movements as appropriate as the movements of those on the floor. If the groups are changed so that each child has frequent opportunities to try every type of activity, all will have an equal chance to profit by these rhythmic experiences.

(3) INDIVIDUAL RESPONSES

Some children are natural followers and respond accurately and well to music while they are in a group where they can observe others. If each pupil is encouraged occasionally to perform by himself, very briefly, it will be possible to make sure that his correct response comes from listening as well as from a musical feeling for the rhythm, and not from imitation of his neighbor.

Children who do not respond accurately to the rhythm of the music, either alone or in groups, should not be classed as deficient in rhythmic sense. It is probable that they need further experience with simple rhythms adjusted to their natural, individual speed of movement as suggested in Chapter I, p. 13, before they will be able to respond accurately to these changing rhythms at the tempo set by the teacher or by other members of the class.

B. CHOICE OF MUSIC

The music for these activities should clearly suggest the change from one natural rhythm to another. It may indicate such changes as

from walking to running to walking,
from walking to skipping to running,
from skipping to walking to running,

or any other combination which seems to promise most effective results. The music selected should follow closely the rhythm patterns suggested on pages 25 - 33, which are associated with walking, skipping and running. The selections at the end of this Chapter (pp. 42 - 48) are presented so that each page provides a contrasting series of rhythms suitable for use together in whatever order seems most desirable: numbers 1 - 2 - 3; 3 - 1 - 2; 2 - 1 - 3, etc. The music given on pages 25 - 33 can also be used in connection with the work of Chapter III, and may be played in a variety of rhythmic sequences.

It has been suggested previously that improvisations or adaptations by the teacher will provide a wealth of additional musical material. The ideas expressed on pages 33 - 36 can also be followed with the music presented in this chapter.

C. RHYTHM INSTRUMENTS

It has already been stated on page 36 that sometimes it is desirable for the teacher to use a hand drum or some similar rhythm instrument in place of the piano to sound the rhythmic patterns for walking, skipping, or running. The change from one rhythm to another can be accomplished smoothly and speedily on such an instrument and provides a variety of experiences for the class. The rhythmic patterns of the piano selections included in Chapter II, and those given in this chapter, will furnish suggestions for different sequences for drum rhythms. It is important that each individual rhythm be continued for at least the equivilent of eight measures of music in order to allow all the children enough time to become adjusted to one rhythm before a change takes place.

(1) USE OF INSTRUMENTS

Use of rhythm instruments by the children themselves to produce the contrasting rhythmic patterns, and also as an activity for recreational periods and an experience for out-of-school hours, should be encouraged. Some children may be found who learn to co-ordinate their muscles in accurate rhythmic response through the playing of such instruments when they have not yet learned to do so through use of the feet or other bodily motion.

However, the same warning as was made in this connection, on page 36, is repeated here: only those who are capable of producing a clear and accurate rhythmic pattern on an instrument should be permitted to provide the rhythm for the class to follow. The time of the entire group will be wasted and no real purpose served if the period is spent in allowing individuals who are retarded in their rhythmic development to experiment with the class.

(2) VARIED ACTIVITIES

It is possible to develop many varied activities which will increase the power of discrimination in recognizing and responding to changing rhythms through the use of several instruments, each of which is chosen for one particular rhythm such as walking, skipping, or running. For example, the large drum may be used for the walking rhythm; the small drum or the triangle for running; the tambourine or gourd rattle for skipping.

Some possible activities are described in this connection for the assistance of the teacher.

(a) The instruments are distributed to some of the children for use with appropriate rhythms as suggested in the preceding paragraphs. The teacher plays a succession of different rhythms on the piano. Part of the class responds through movement. At the same time those having instruments listen carefully, each person playing when the music suggests his instrument, and only then. When the piano indicates walking, the large drum plays with it; when skipping is suggested the tambourine or gourd rattle takes its turn; when a running rhythm is heard the triangle or small drum plays an accompaniment with it.

(b) A complete set of rhythm band instruments can be used in much the same way. The instruments that rattle or jingle when shaken are best for skipping: tambourines, rattles, shakers, jingle bells, castanets, clogs, etc. The tinkling instruments are used for running: triangles, cymbals struck very lightly, orchestra bells, etc. Heavier percussion instruments are used for walking: drums, rhythm sticks, wood blocks, tom-toms, guiros, cabassas, etc. Each group plays only when music containing its special rhythmic pattern is heard.

(c) Three instruments are distributed. One should be suitable for walking, one for running, and one for skipping. The three players take turns playing their rhythmic patterns while the class responds. This provides an opportunity for creative activity by the children who have good co-ordination and feeling for rhythm, and at the same time keeps the entire class engaged in an active experience. The instrumental players frequently acquire a surprising degree of skill in organizing their playing so as to go smoothly and evenly from one rhythm to another.

(3) MUSICAL SELECTIONS

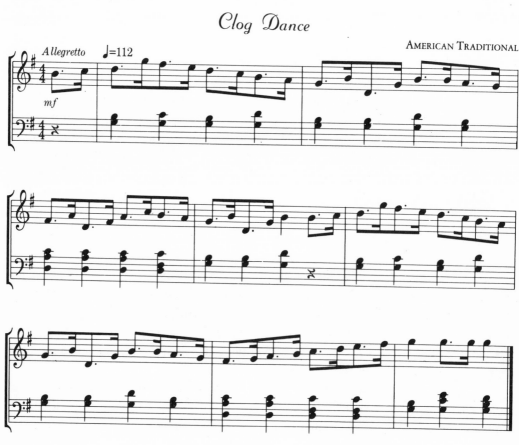

Clog Dance

AMERICAN TRADITIONAL

Hungarian Folk Tune

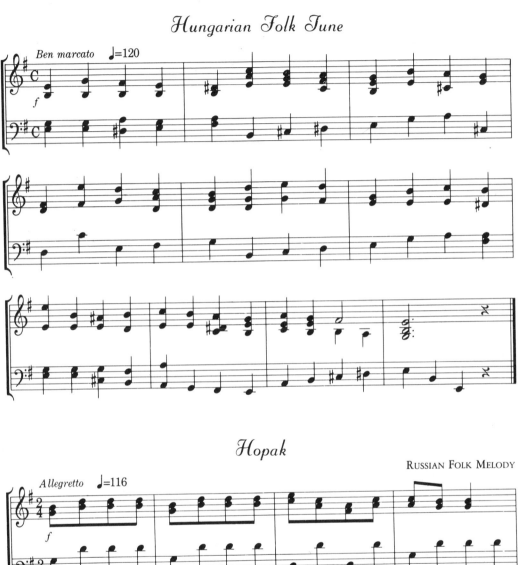

Hopak

RUSSIAN FOLK MELODY

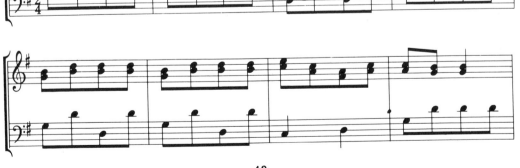

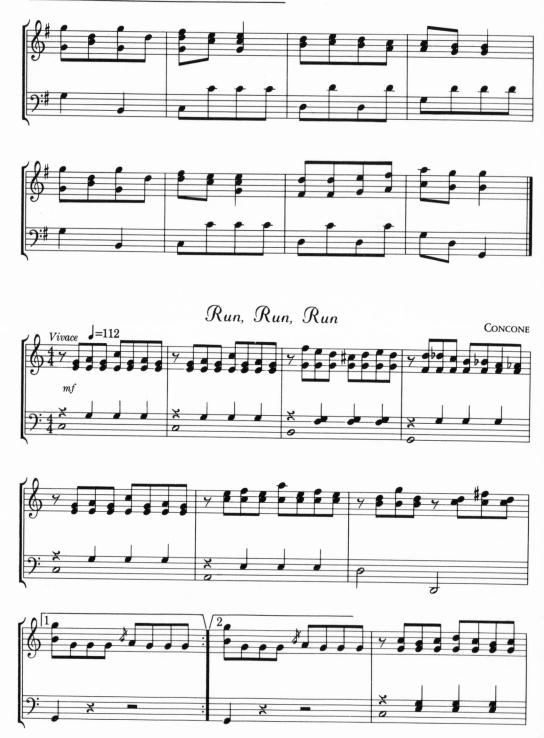

Run, Run, Run

CONCONE

Money Musk

SCOTCH FOLK MELODY

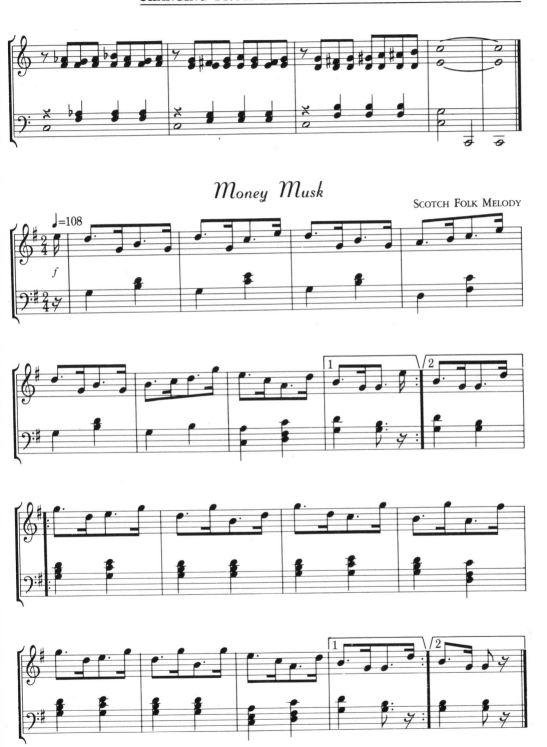

Little Man in a Fix

SWEDISH FOLK MELODY

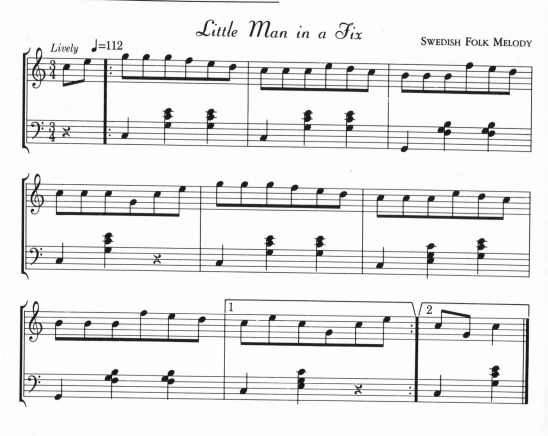

The Secret

L. GAUTIER

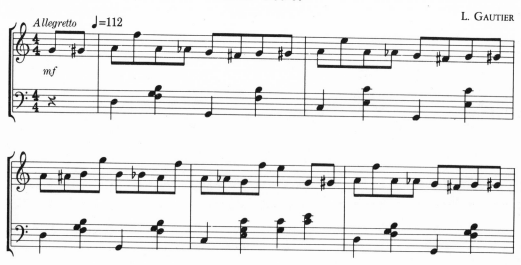

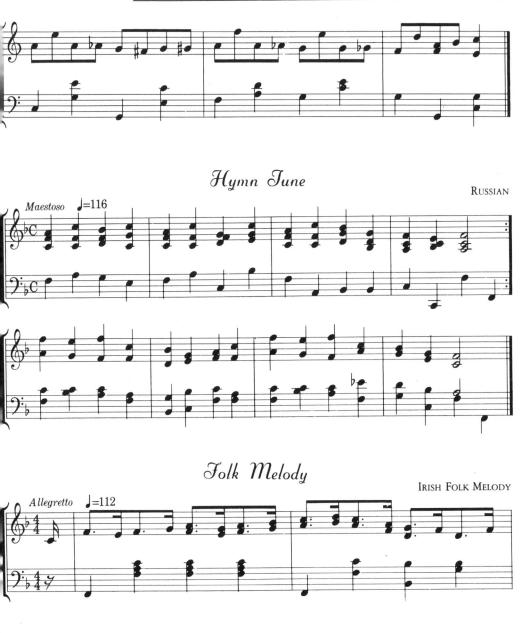

Hymn Tune

RUSSIAN

Maestoso ♩=116

Folk Melody

IRISH FOLK MELODY

Allegretto ♩=112

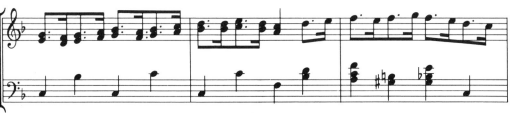

47

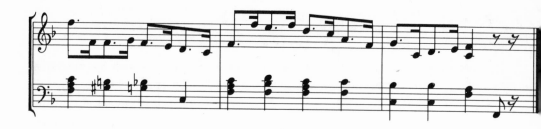

Chapter IV
Phrases in Music

It is important that the term "phrase" as used in connection with the activities of this and succeeding chapters be clearly understood. Because of their different viewpoints, the music educator and the theorist usually give different definitions to this word. For example, the song "Swinging in the Willow" contains eight measures of music distributed on four staves of two measures each. According to strictly formal analysis there are two phases in the song, each phrase having four measures. Some authorities call these phrases the antecedent and the consequent.

A small child, however, usually feels a shorter musical unit than this in his first experience with phrasing. For this reason it has become the practice in music books for children to divide the full phrase into two sections, each of which contains only two measures. Wherever possible, each phrase section is put on a separate staff. The term "phrase" referring to one of these short sections or lines is now quite generally accepted by music educators.

Swinging in the Willow (Listen and Sing, p. 17)

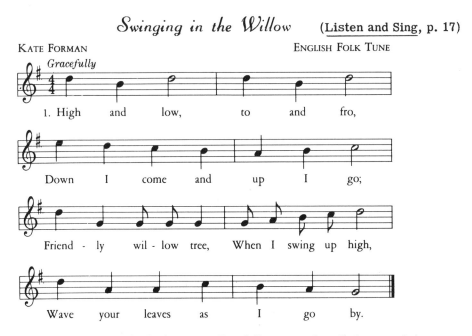

KATE FORMAN ENGLISH FOLK TUNE

Gracefully

1. High and low, to and fro,

Down I come and up I go;

Friend - ly wil - low tree, When I swing up high,

Wave your leaves as I go by.

All individuals will not feel phrase units of the same length in a certain song. The teacher should not feel undue concern if the children feel phrases differently from the way she feels them. The pupil may feel the phrase to be only one half as

49

long, or he may feel it to be twice as long as the teacher does. For instance, in a short song such as "Round the Pear Tree" some children may feel the first two staves (four measures) as the first phrase, and the teacher should accept their response as satisfactory.

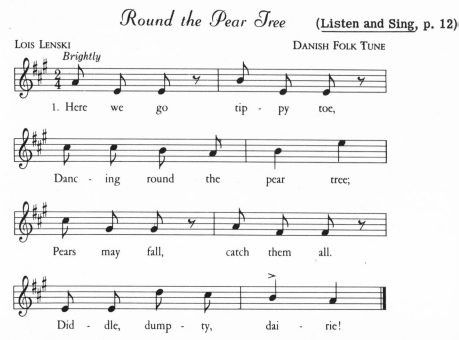

Round the Pear Tree   (Listen and Sing, p. 12)

Lois Lenski   Danish Folk Tune

1. Here we go tip - py toe,

Danc - ing round the pear tree;

Pears may fall, catch them all.

Did - dle, dump - ty, dai - rie!

Meticulous insistence upon analysis of the music for correct divisions into phrases of a certain definite length is not desirable at this point. If the children can feel as they sing, play and listen, that the music is divided into parts, that "one part" ends here, another "part" begins there, our objective will have been reached in so far as feeling for the phrase unit is concerned. Much experience of the type offered by the activities described in this chapter will lead not only to an increase in the child's consciousness of phrase balance and beauty, but also to a maturing of his conception of what constitutes the musical phrase.

A. PROCEDURE

(1) UNDERSTANDING OF PHRASES IN SONGS

The meaning of the term <u>phrase</u> in a song will be familiar to children who have learned a large number of rote songs. The wise teacher, when teaching rote songs in the lower grades, will introduce the word <u>phrase</u> so naturally and so incidentally that the children will learn the meaning with little or no explanation.

She may say, "I'll sing the first <u>phrase</u> again." "Who would like to sing this <u>phrase</u> after me?" Or while teaching a song including a repeated refrain such as "Chickadee" she may suggest, "Let's see how many boys and girls can sing the phrase 'Sing for me, Chickadee' every time it appears, while I sing the rest of the song." In this way, without making any special effort, the children absorb the significance of the word <u>phrase</u> as applied to rote songs they are learning to sing.

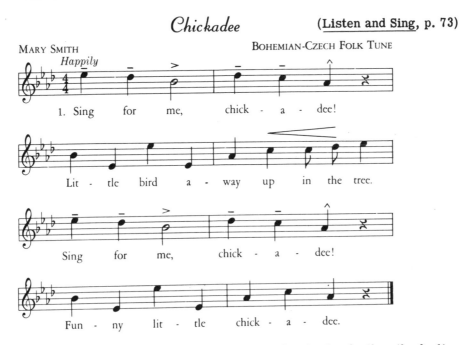

Chickadee   <u>(Listen and Sing, p. 73)</u>

MARY SMITH   BOHEMIAN-CZECH FOLK TUNE

There are several activities which will assist in developing further the feeling for the phrases in a song:

(a) The teacher may sing a phrase from a very familiar song, using a neutral syllable. Then she may ask the class or one pupil to sing the words that belong to this phrase. "Has anyone heard this tune before?" "Who can sing it back to me using the words?" "What are the words to the next phrase in the song?"

(b) Four children may be chosen to stand before the class and sing a familiar four-phrase song, such as "Pay with a Smile." One child is assigned to sing the first phrase, another the second, and so on. Or the song may be sung by four rows or four table groups, each group chosen to sing a certain phrase. The teacher gives the pitch and signal for starting the first phrase, and then the children sing the song without making any breaks or stops between the phrases. After a few songs have been sung in this manner the teacher should be careful to give no indication to the different rows or individuals as to when they should begin to sing or should stop singing. The song should always be sung smoothly with no break in its continuity, a complete, artistic unit, even when different individuals or groups are singing different phrases.

Pay with a Smile (Rhythms and Rimes, p. 73)

After the original by
ETHEL CROWNINSHIELD

IRISH FOLK SONG

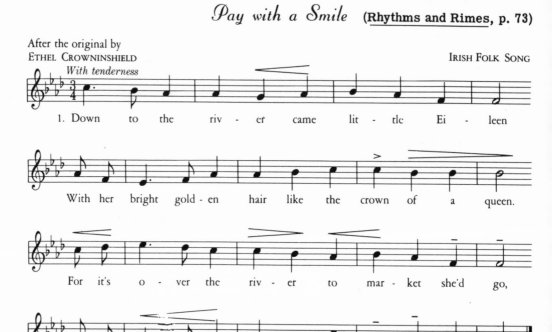

1. Down to the riv - er came lit - tle Ei - leen
With her bright gold - en hair like the crown of a queen.
For it's o - ver the riv - er to mar - ket she'd go,
And she'll bring back a bun - ny that's white as the snow.

(c) Children enjoy the experience of alternating the singing of words and neutral syllables on different phrases. It adds variety. When singing a familiar song, words may be used with the first phrase, "loo" with the second, words with the third, and "tah" or some other syllable with the fourth. Or the procedure may be varied by having the children sing the first phrase with words, the second phrase silently to themselves, the third phrase aloud, and so on to the conclusion of the song. This requires silent singing of the melody, and is excellent training in thinking melody and rhythm.

These same practices may also be used with individuals and smaller groups of children. Individual singing of phrases is often very revealing to a teacher; it provides an opportunity to hear the different pupils clearly and briefly, and to discover weaknesses and correct them. Children may be found who sing the tune incorrectly, sing wrong words or mispronounce other words, do not know the words, or have bad vocal habits.

(d) After a good deal of experience with phrases in familiar songs, the children may be requested to listen for the phrases in new songs. For example, the teacher sings a song which the class has not heard previously. After some discussion the teacher may ask the pupils to close their eyes, listen to the song once more, and raise their hands at the end of each phrase. Or they may be asked to count the phrases. Afterwards the class can learn the song phrasewise as the teacher sings, or they may learn it by singing the repeated phrases while she sings the whole song until all of it is entirely familiar.

B. MOVEMENT

(1) RESPONSE TO PHRASES IN SONGS SUNG AND MUSIC HEARD

In addition to understanding the phrases in the songs they sing, children should be led to notice that, even when there are no words, the music seems to be divided into parts; in other words, "here one part of the melody ends" and "here another part begins." Soon they will begin to realize that these parts sound like phrases and are called phrases. Through response by physical movement to these phrases (either in songs or in instrumental music) they will develop a clearer and more satisfying understanding of the music. The following activities are suggested to provide this experience:

(a) The teacher plays a familiar selection on either the piano or the phonograph. It may be a selection that has been used in one of the preceding lessons, such as "Hopak" on page 43. It is important that the phrases in the selection be short and clearly defined. The children may be asked to close their eyes as they listen to the music, and to raise their hands at the end of each phrase. They should be able to tell how many phrases there are in the composition.

(b) The children, with eyes closed as they sing or listen to music such as is included at the end of this chapter, raise their arms slowly in an outward-upward circular motion to show the rise of the phrase, and lower the arms gradually to show the fall of the phrase, touching the fingers of both hands in front of the body as the phrase ends.

During this activity the children will develop a fuller, freer feeling for the phrase if they stand, "take distance" from each other by describing an arc with the arms in order to be sure they are far enough apart, and then close their eyes and mark the phrases, using the arms widely and freely. They will also gradually learn to co-ordinate their breathing with the rise and fall of the phrase line as they indicate this by the movement of the arms. When this type of phrasing activity is used with songs, smoother, more sustained, and more artistic singing results.

53

(c) With some instrumental selections the children may "play the violin" on every other phrase and "rest" (listen, not play) on the alternate phrases. This experience may be varied by having one row "play" the first phrase, the next row the second phrase, and so on to the end of the selection.

It is usually wise to have the children close their eyes as they mark the phrases, so that the teacher can observe how each individual feels the phrases when he is not influenced by what his neighbor is doing. Sometimes, however, the experience will be greatly intensified if the class phrases while the teacher or a leader chosen from the group directs and defines the phrase pattern.

(2) PHRASING WITH RHYTHM INSTRUMENTS

After many successful experiences with sensing phrases in songs and instrumental music, the rhythm band (or selected rhythm instruments) may be used as a medium for the further development and expression of the child's feeling for the phrase. Not all groups will have the same instruments, but in general most classes will have available instruments that can be divided into families or choirs. These may be the rattle-jingle group, the tinkler group, and the percussion group, as was suggested on page 41.

It has been suggested in Chapter III that each of these different groups play whenever a certain rhythm is heard. This discrimination can now be carried further. For example, after listening to a song or instrumental piece and showing the phrases by rhythmic movement, as was suggested earlier in this chapter, the children may decide which family of instruments fits each phrase; the jinglers may play the first phrase, the tinklers the second, the percussions the third, while all play together on the fourth. Or, in case of a selection in which a repeated refrain or phrase occurs ("Chickadee," p. 51) children will frequently choose to have the same group of instruments play each time the repeated phrase occurs, and a different group play on the alternate phrases.

(3) CREATIVE PHRASING

Children enjoy making up their own games for showing phrase feeling. After the teacher has led the way with some of the activities suggested in previous paragraphs, the children will be familiar with the idea of phrasewise response. From now on members of the class should be encouraged to invent activities which will show that they sense the phrases in the music.

It will be of interest to teachers to know some of the simple phrase responses that have been created by children. One boy, as a march was being played, stepped in one direction during the first phrase, and at the beginning of the second phrase executed an "about face" and marched in the opposite direction. He continued in this fashion to the end of the music. During the playing of music for running, four boys wanted to show the class a new phrase game. The first boy started running on the first phrase, the second boy on the second phrase, and so on. Later they established correct distances from one another and ran in relays, each spacing his steps and timing himself so that just at the end of his phrase he reached the next runner and started him on his way. At another time, music suggesting the dancing of fairies was played. The girl who volunteered to show the class the phrases in the music danced lightly around the front of the room during the first phrase, and on the second phrase she turned around and around on tiptoe in one spot. She alternated phrasewise in this way throughout the entire selection. One class chose a leader who directed the phrasing by pointing, as each new phrase started, to a different group or row of children. This pupil-leader stood at the front of the room and made a special movement to fit the music of each phrase, and the group designated for that phrase imitated his motions.

The resourceful class and the class where wholesome self-expression has been encouraged will find many ways of revealing a feeling for the mood as well as the length of the phrase.

(4) SIMULTANEOUS ACTIVITIES

The activities suggested in Chapters V and VI may be carried on simultaneously with the phrasing activities of this chapter. The teacher should not defer the introduction of these additional activities until all of these phrasing experiences can be carried on successfully.

C. MUSIC FOR PHRASING ACTIVITIES

(1) SONGS

Most of the songs children sing in class will provide ideal material for their phrasing activities. Suggestions with regard to the phrases in songs are given in the first section of this chapter.

(2) PIANO MUSIC

For some of the activities suggested in other chapters of this book, the choice of music to be sung or played is limited to that which includes only certain kinds of measure or note values. There are no such limitations on the music to be used for phrasing. Music in all kinds of different measures and with all kinds of note values may be used. However, care should be taken:

(a) To select music in which the phrase is short enough to match the child's span of attention.

(b) To play the music with artistic phrasing.

In addition to the music included at the end of this chapter, many selections for these activities of phrase sensing are to be found in "Play a Tune" of The World of Music series. The classified contents on pages 4-6 presents titles of many instrumental selections especially valuable for experiences in phrasing.

(3) PHONOGRAPH RECORDS

Many compositions appropriate for use with the activities of this chapter, including some already suggested, are available on phonograph records. The interested teacher should consult educational record catalogs or the educational departments of the various phonograph companies for recommended lists of recordings.

Cradle Song

MISKA HAUSER

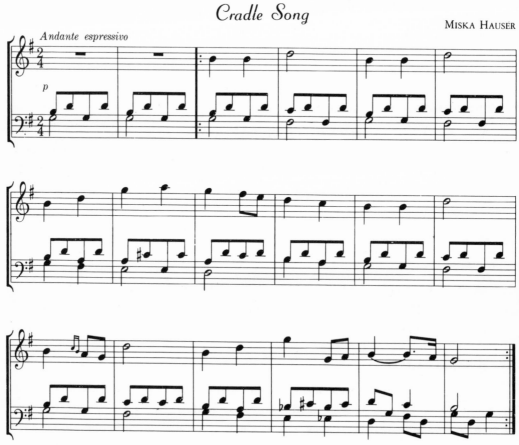

An Alexis

J. N. HUMMEL

Minuet (Don Juan)

W. A. MOZART

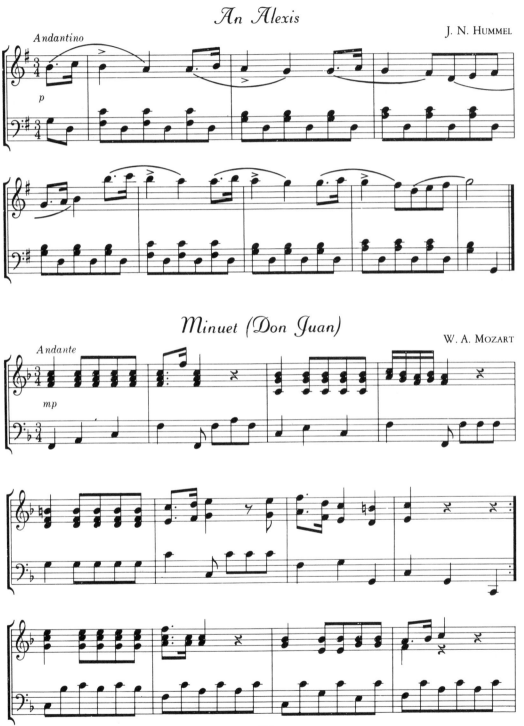

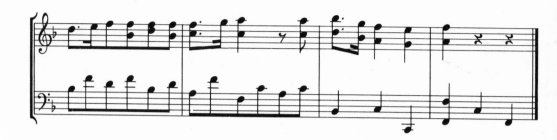

Chapter V
Response to Notes
Longer than Walking Notes

The activities outlined in this chapter can be successfully carried on at the same time as those suggested in Chapter IV. Before proceeding with these activities the children should be very familiar with music that suggests walking, running and skipping, so that they can recognize by ear the note combinations which suggest these movements, and show their recognition through rhythmic movement.

A. PROCEDURE

(1) DISCOVERING THE LONGER NOTES

The teacher plays "Turkish Folk Tune" or "German Folk Tune" or some similar selection that begins with walking or quarter notes and later changes to half, dotted half or whole notes. While the teacher plays, pupils remain seated, listening and ready to tell which of the three familiar movements the music indicates: walk, run, or skip. These two selections are not for floor activity. They are for recognition through listening, not stepping.

Turkish Folk Tune
(Tuning Up, p. 79)

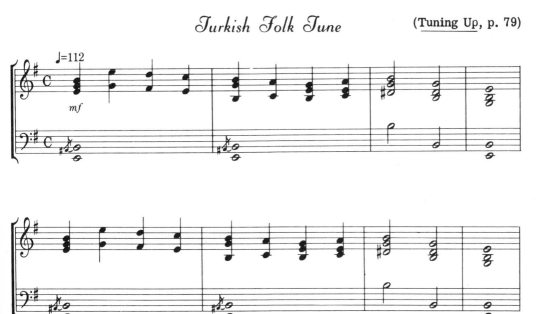

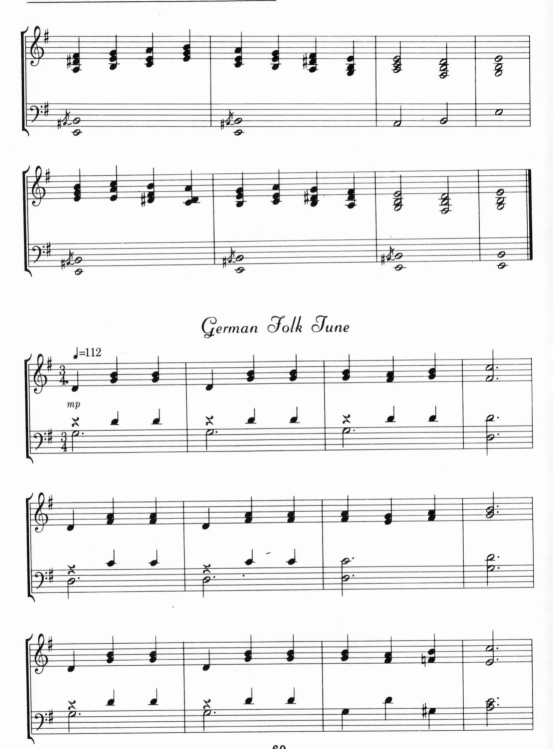

German Folk Tune

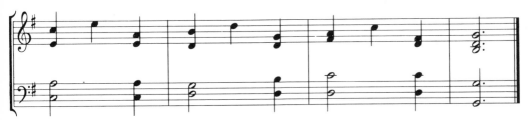

Since the children hear the quarter notes first, they are likely to identify the music as walking music. They listen again while the first eight measures are played, to try to discover any notes that are not walking notes. Someone hears notes that are longer than walking notes. Again, listening to the music, the children "walk" with their arms (swinging the arms down on each quarter note), as they are accustomed to do when demonstrating the walking rhythm at their seats. In this way they try to discover how many steps, or arm swings, they make to each of these longer notes. In the "Turkish Folk Tune" they will find that for some notes the arm moves downward twice, for other notes four times. In the "German Folk Tune" they will find that some notes require three downward arm swings.

For these introductory lessons the teacher and pupils can refer to half notes as two-beat notes, to dotted half notes as three-beat notes, and to whole notes as four-beat notes. As soon as the longer notes have been discovered by ear the class is ready to concentrate on these three new kinds of notes with rhythmic response on the floor.

(2) RESPONSE: RHYTHMIC MOVEMENT TO MUSIC IN WHICH ONLY ONE KIND OF LONGER NOTE IS HEARD

In connection with all the following activities it is often impossible or undesirable to have the entire class respond on the floor at the same time. The pupils who remain at their seats will participate by keeping time as they listen to the music, usually by swinging their arms. In this way they are constantly responding to the rhythm of the music and will be able to join or take the place of the group on the floor easily at any time. Children get an understanding of these activities best by first watching the performance of someone else. The group will grasp the idea quickly if there is a demonstration by the teacher or by a group of pupils from a higher grade. Each selection heard contains only one kind of note in the right-hand-melody line. When the music is first played the class listens, swings arms, and recognizes the music as being made up of two-beat, three-beat, or four-beat notes, as the case may be. Then the teacher or demonstration group responds as follows:

61

LEARNING MUSIC THROUGH RHYTHM

(a) ♩ If the music contains two-beat or half notes, the pupils stand and swing the arms steadily, "one, two, down, down," until the feeling for the two-beat note is well established. Then they move, taking one step and only one for each note, meanwhile swinging the arms twice for each note. It is important that the step be taken rhythmically on the first beat of each note. In these illustrations the right hand is to be played forte; the left hand, piano.

Sacred Melody

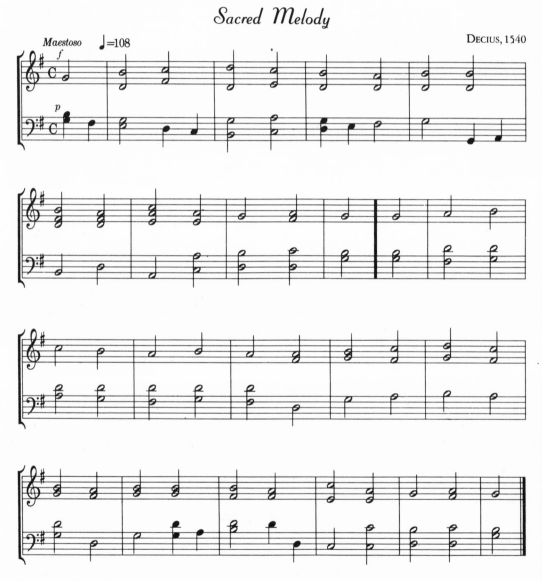

DECIUS, 1540

Maestoso ♩=108

62

Chorale

GERMAN, 1558

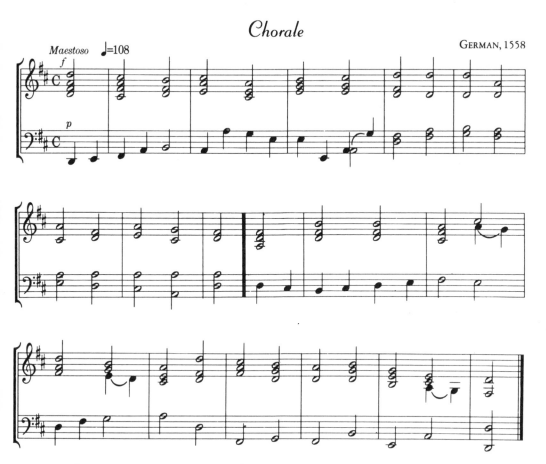

(b) ♩. When a succession of three-beat or dotted half notes is played, the arms swing downward three times for each note, but <u>only one</u> step is taken for each note and, as before, this occurs on the <u>first</u> beat of the note.

Intermezzo Russe

FRANKE

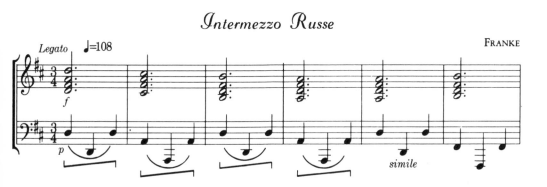

63

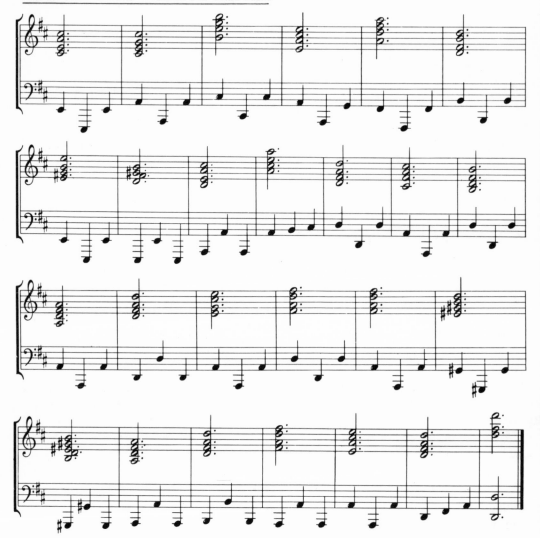

(c) ◦ When four-beat, or whole, notes are heard, the arms swing downward four times for each note, but the foot takes just <u>one</u> step forward for each note and that step is taken on the first beat.

Adoremus te

PALESTRINA

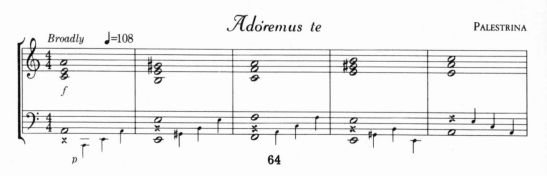

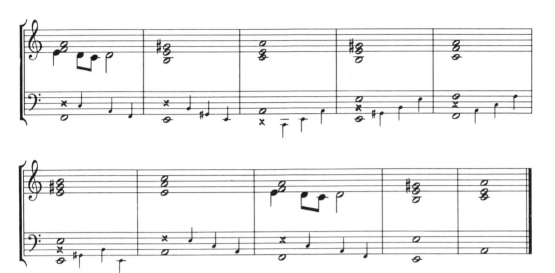

As soon as the pupils understand these responses for the various note values as they are demonstrated, they are ready to try the activities for themselves. A small group of six or eight children stand in single file or in a large circle. As the teacher begins to play, the children <u>listen</u> to a few measures, keeping time with a downward sweep of the forearm, just as they did at their seats. When they are sure of the length of the notes they are hearing, the teacher gives the signal and they begin to take a step for each note, as already outlined.

It is important that each musical selection used for these first activities contain only one type of note, so that the children can have plenty of experience with that note and its significance, recognizing it, and acquiring the necessary muscular control to respons to it rhythmically. The music which has been presented in this chapter provides the necessary material for carefully organized preliminary experience of this kind. After many opportunities have been given to insure a good degree of success in making these responses, music which includes a combination of note values may be used.

(3) RESPONSES TO MUSIC INCLUDING HALF NOTES, DOTTED HALF NOTES, AND WHOLE NOTES IN ANY ORDER

The preceding responses, as a rule, are soon mastered, and the children next demonstrate that they recognize the change when the music moves smoothly from one kind of note to another. They stand in single file as before, ready to respond rhythmically by swinging arms and stepping notes. Without intimating that something new is to be introduced, the teacher plays one of the improvisations which follow. As the music changes from one note value to another, the pupils sense that something is different and their initial response no longer fits. Those who are listening carefully to the music and who have a well-developed rhythmic feeling solve the problem quickly by changing their rhythmic action to fit the new kind of note. The others gradually acquire this ability through experience.

In the improvisations either eight or sixteen measures of one kind of note are presented before change to another note value occurs. This is done so that the children may have ample time to adjust themselves to each in turn. Care must be taken that the tempo of the beat does not change, even though the note values do. A change in tempo will not only call attention to the change in note values, but will also complicate the change in response which members of the class are making.

Improvisation 1[1]

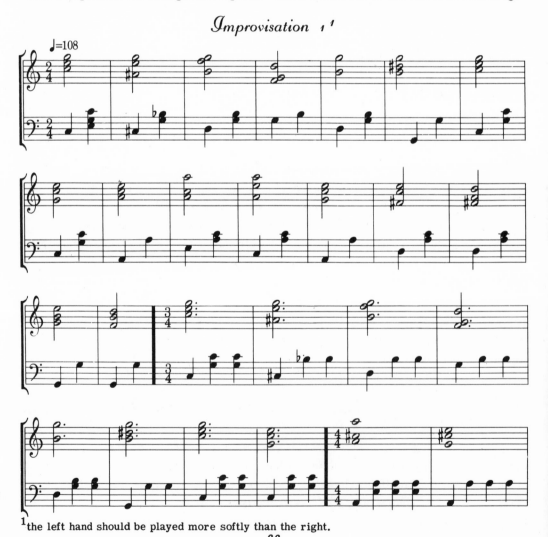

[1]the left hand should be played more softly than the right.

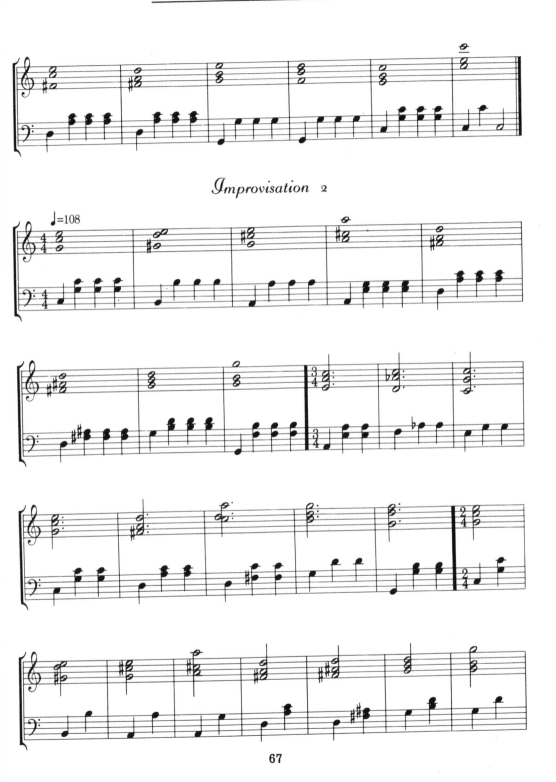

Improvisation 2

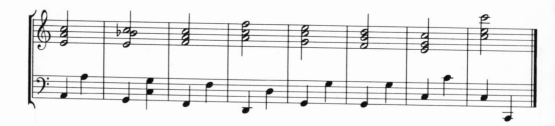

B. CHOICE OF MUSIC FOR STUDY OF THESE LONGER NOTES

The selections included in this chapter have been chosen to meet the requirements which are listed in the paragraphs which follow. In all the music used for
these activities, any quarter notes in the bass or in the harmonic accompaniment
should be played more softly than the melody, in fact, just loudly enough to be
heard, for the sake of continuous rhythmic movement.

(1) HALF NOTES

Music used to develop an understanding of the half note should be in 2/4 or
4/4 measure, consisting almost entirely of half notes in the right-hand-melody
line.

(2) DOTTED HALF NOTES

Music for this experience with dotted half notes should be in 3/4 measure.
There should be little else in the right-hand-melody line than dotted half notes.

(3) WHOLE NOTES

For experience with whole notes the music should be in 4/4 measure, or
common time (C), and should consist almost entirely of whole notes in the right-
hand-melody line.

C. ADAPTING MUSIC

The teacher can provide a greater variety of music for the activities presented in this chapter by improvising or by adapting some of the music, to make it
follow a certain rhythmic pattern. The suggestions which follow may help any
teacher who has had little experience with the keyboard.

(1) In "Improvisation 1" the last eight measures may be changed from 4/4 to
2/4 measure. The whole notes in the right hand may be changed to half notes, and

the first two beats of the left-hand accompaniment only may be used, omitting the chords for the third and fourth beats, thus:

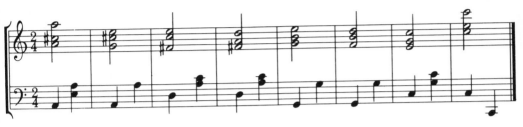

The same procedure may be used to change the first eight measures in "Improvisation 2" from 4/4 to 2/4 measure, half notes taking the place of whole notes in the right hand, and the chords or notes on the third and fourth beats in the left-hand accompaniment being omitted.

(2) Another possibility is to play the first eight measures of "Improvisation 1" in 4/4 rather than 2/4 measure. This will necessitate the substitution of whole notes for half notes in the right hand, and two repetitions of the chord or note on the second beat in the left-hand accompaniment, thus:

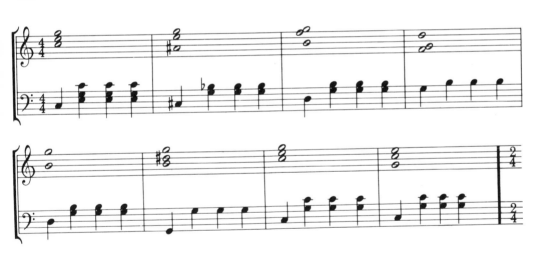

This eight-measure period will provide enough music for adequate experience with whole notes for most groups, and will be more practical than to continue with whole notes for the entire sixteen measures.

(3) The change to or from the dotted half note can be accomplished in the same way. Such changes permit greater variety, and if such variations are used the thirty-two measures of "Improvisation 1" can produce more effective results. Here is one possibility:

69

measures 1 - 8   2/4 measure with ♩

measures 9 - 16   3/4 measure with ♩

measures 17 - 24 4/4 measure with ○

measures 25 - 32 2/4 measure with ♩

Numerous other similar changes will provide a succession of interesting experiences with both "Improvisation 1" and "Improvisation 2." The majority of classes will grasp the activities of this chapter quickly. Unless a class needs further experience with these note values, improvisations 1 and 2 should be sufficient music material.

D. RHYTHMIC NOTATION

Some teachers prefer to introduce the notation of these notes at the same time that pupils are responding to them. While good results can sometimes be accomplished by so doing, it is recommended that much experience in physical movement precede the presentation of the notation. This accords with the principle the thing before the sign. Therefore the association of these rhythms with their notation is not introduced until Chapter VIII.

E. USE OF RHYTHM INSTRUMENTS

Some rhythm instruments can be used for additional experience with these longer notes. The gong is especially effective for giving a clearer understanding of the long notes and their two-beat, three-beat, or four-beat length. It is also possible to use the drum, which, although it has no means of sustaining the tone for the full value of the note, if used with the piano or voice can do much to stress the length of each note by emphasizing the beginning of the note. The gong or drum can be struck on the first beat of the long note, and the player then indicates the length of the note by one free (silent) swing of the arm away from the instrument for each additional beat. Thus a ♩ would be played strike, swing; ○ would be strike, swing, swing, swing.

Chapter VI
Responses to Music
with Varied Rhythmic Note Patterns

Thus far the pupils have had experience with rhythmic patterns made up of the following notes:

Walking ♩ ♩ ♩ ♩   Two-beat notes 𝅗𝅥 𝅗𝅥

Running ♫♫ ♫♫   Three-beat notes 𝅗𝅥. 𝅗𝅥.

Skipping ♪. ♫♪. ♪. ♫♪. ♪   Four-beat notes 𝅝 𝅝

They have recognized and responded to music in which the rhythm changes from one pattern to another: walking to running to skipping; running to walking to skipping, and so on. They have also recognized and responded to music in which variations in the rhythmic pattern follow a change in the value or length of the predominating note, a half note, a dotted half, or a whole note.

In this chapter the music presented will involve changes from any one of the six patterns listed above to any other.

A. IMPORTANCE OF PREVIOUS EXPERIENCE

Before commencing the activities presented on these pages, it is essential that the children should have a great many successful associations with all of the experiences which have been outlined in the preceding chapters. If the rhythmic sense and understanding have been allowed to develop at a normal, easy pace, the pupils will approach any new problem in a relaxed, confident way that insures success. If, however, the children have been pushed ahead too rapidly by a teacher whose chief anxiety is to cover the ground quickly, they will be nervous and hurried and unable to acquire the understanding, muscular control, and musical feeling necessary to make these musical activities successful and enjoyable.

B. PROCEDURE

In Chapters III and V suggestions and directions are given for responding to music in which the basic rhythms are changed. If these ideas have been thoroughly developed, the new experiences suggested in this chapter will not be entirely strange, and should present no serious difficulties.

71

LEARNING MUSIC THROUGH RHYTHM

The children who are to respond on the floor are asked to line up in single file, ready for the music to begin. They already know these suggestions for procedure:

(1) They must first listen to a few measures in order to <u>hear</u> what rhythmic movement is suggested by the music.

(2) As soon as they discover what the music is telling them, they must be ready for the signal to begin their individual responses by rhythmic <u>movement</u>.

(3) While they respond, they must be listening for possible rhythmic changes in the music.

(4) As soon as they recognize any change in the music they must immediately alter their movements to fit the new rhythm.

The teacher plays the following group of three pieces in sequence:

Mountain March

NORWEGIAN FOLK DANCE

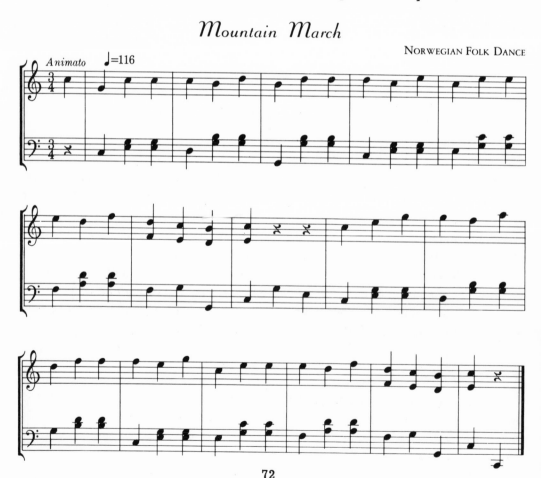

72

Excerpt from "Melody"

THOMÉ

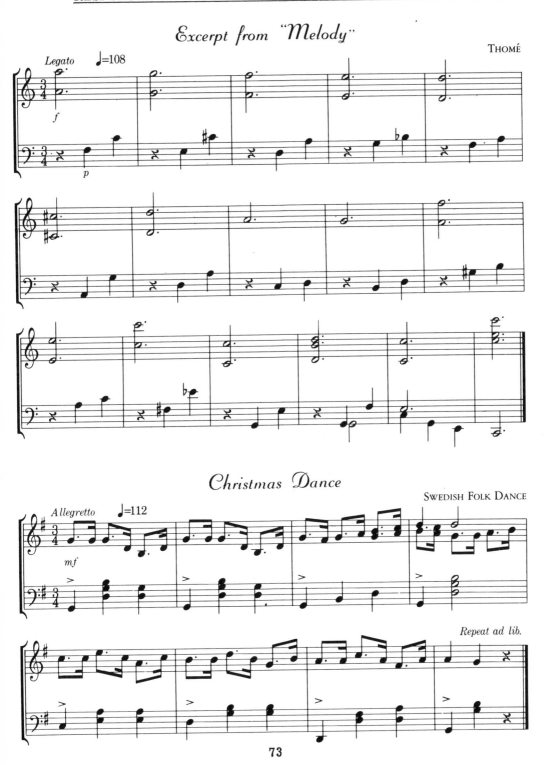

Christmas Dance

SWEDISH FOLK DANCE

Repeat ad lib.

LEARNING MUSIC THROUGH RHYTHM

The progress from one kind of music to another must be made smoothly and without a halt or break to reveal the change in rhythm. The children as they listen will synchronize their rhythmic movements.

Since it is not usually practical to have all the members of the class make their responses on the floor at the same time, those remaining in their seats may make their rhythmic responses by arm movements, as has been suggested in previous chapters.

C. MUSIC FOR EXPERIENCE WITH CHANGING RHYTHMS

Two additional groups, each including three instrumental pieces, are presented here in sequence. These pieces are arranged for the activities described in this chapter. If possible, the teacher will find it desirable to play other combinations of rhythms, examples such as may be found in Play a Tune, or may even improvise them.

It is desirable, if printed scores are used, that the teacher play from memory as much as possible, since then undivided attention may be given to the pupils and to their responses. Suggestions for improvisation are given on pages · 33, 66, and 69. Additional material may be made available by alternating some of the selections in Chapters II and III with some of those presented in Chapter V.

The musical selections which are appropriate for each rhythmic change should be from eight to sixteen measures long, depending upon the kind of measure and the time necessary for children to change from one type of response to another. Since quarter notes are most frequently used as the "beat" notes, they set the tempo or rate of speed better than other notes. Therefore it is suggested that the rhythmic sequences always change from ♪ to ♩ and not from ♩ or ♪ to ♩. However, it is possible to change satisfactorily from the longer notes such as ♩., ♩, 𝅝 to skips and runs, without the quarter note (♩) coming in between.

Melody

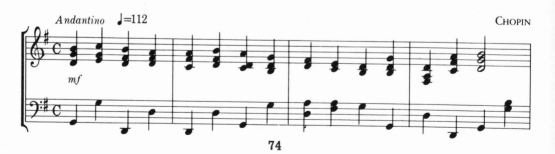

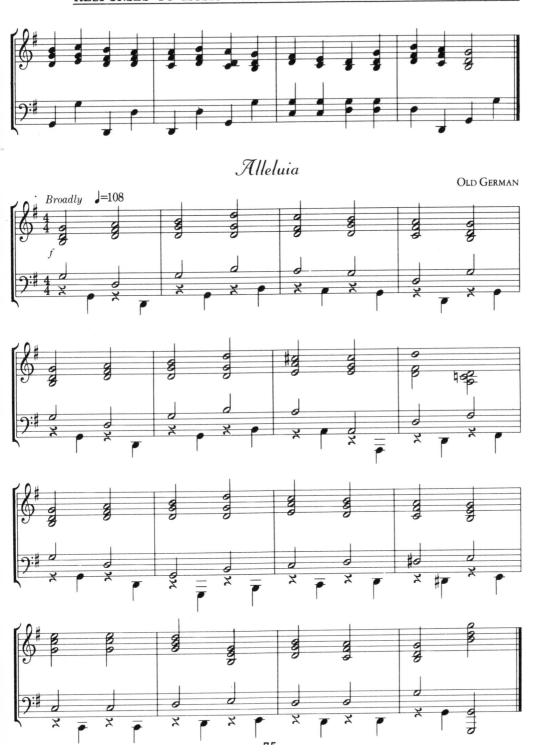

Alleluia

OLD GERMAN

Chord Study

KALKBRENNER

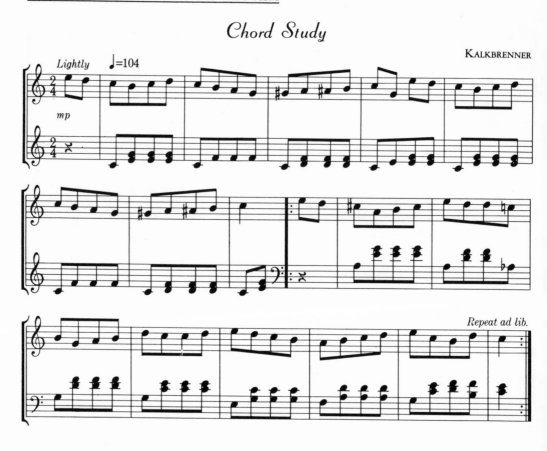

Highland Schottische

SCOTCH

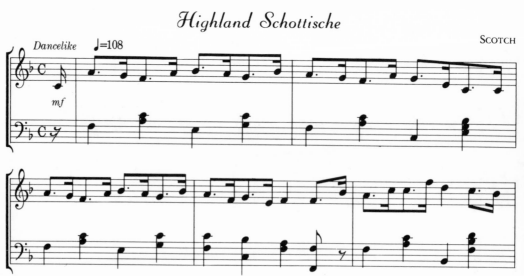

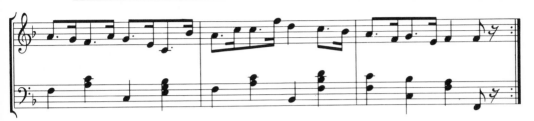

Folk Tune

GERMAN

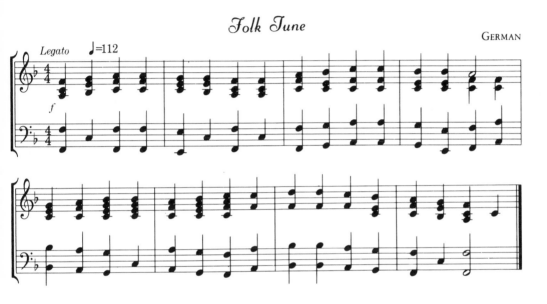

Descant "There's Music in the Air"

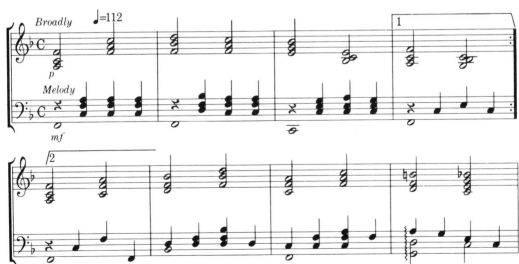

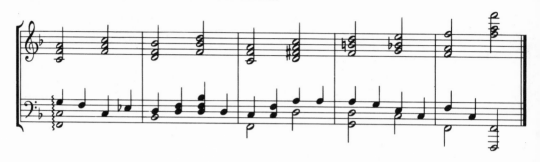

Chapter VII
Responses to Like and Unlike Phrases

Up to now children have developed not only an understanding of the musical phrase in songs which they sing and in music they hear, but also an ability to recognize and respond to these phrases. It is extremely important that the group have for a foundation abundant experience in the activities suggested in Chapter IV, and that the majority of the pupils be able to sing melodies well and in tune before starting to carry out any of the ideas which are presented in the succeeding pages.

Observant pupils undoubtedly will have learned to notice early in the rote-song experience that many songs include two or more phrases which are either identical or very similar in melodic and rhythmic patterns. For example, the song "A Modern Cinderella" (Listen and Sing, p. 54) consists of four song phrases. The first and third are exactly alike, while the second and fourth are contrasting phrases; that is, they differ both in melody and rhythm from the first and third. In presenting the activities described in this chapter, the aim is to bring about a consciousness of this phrase repetition, or similarity, on the part of all the children.

A. DISCOVERY OF LIKE AND UNLIKE PHRASES IN FAMILIAR SONGS

Children have become accustomed to recognizing phrases in songs they sing by having different groups or individuals sing the various phrases. (See Chapter IV.) Now as they review a familiar song such as "A Modern Cinderella," each phrase in the song is assigned to a different group of children to sing. One child is appointed to act as judge to decide, by listening, which two or more groups are singing the same melody, and which are singing different melodies.

A Modern Cinderella (Listen and Sing, p. 54)

JEAN BEECHAM   MARY B. BLACK

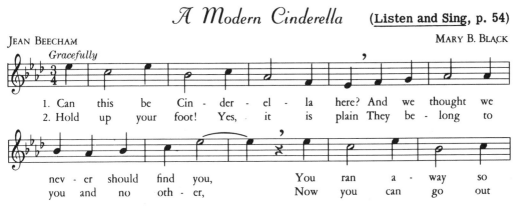

1. Can this be Cin-der-el-la here? And we thought we
2. Hold up your foot! Yes, it is plain They be-long to

nev-er should find you,   You ran a-way so
you and no oth-er,   Now you can go out

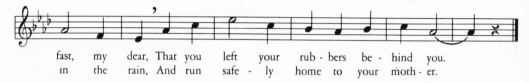

fast,   my   dear, That you   left   your   rub - bers   be - hind   you.
in   the   rain, And run   safe - ly   home   to   your   moth - er.

Using some other familiar four-phrase song which includes a repeated phrase, four children may be chosen to stand before the class, each to sing one phrase of the song, using a neutral syllable. A fifth child may act as the judge who is to decide which of the phrases are alike and which are different.

Various experiences of this type should be continued until the majority of the children easily recognize the like and unlike phrases in the songs they sing. The use of a neutral syllable (loo, tah, etc.) in singing songs for this purpose is highly recommended. The fact that two phrases have two different sets of words will often make it difficult for the child to recognize that the same melody and rhythm are used in both. The neutral syllables allow opportunities for concentrating the attention on the melody and rhythm without the distraction of the changing words.

B. SINGING RESPONSE: LIKE AND UNLIKE PHRASES OF FAMILIAR SONGS

(1) As soon as the children learn by listening that songs may include two or more phrases that are alike, they can begin to make a response which shows these repetitions of melody and rhythm. Sometimes this is done by singing the words to the first phrase of the song and to all other like phrases, but singing neutral syllables to those phrases which are different, or vice versa.

(2) For another type of response, one child or one row of children may sing the first phrase and all other like phrases, while another child or row, or even the entire class, sings all contrasting phrases. Children in intermediate and upper grades will enjoy expressing their recognition of song form by making letter diagrams which use the same letter for repeated phrases such as ABAC or AABC. They will discover that some songs include only two melodies in their four phrases, the first and third being alike and the fourth being a repetition of the second, thus: ABAB.

(3) Through a variety of such activities the pupils will acquire a keen understanding of the repetition and contrast in melody and rhythm that make up a song. Before long some of the more musical members of the class will be noticing that two phrases begin alike, but that they end with slightly different melodic or rhythmic patterns. It is important that the songs used for first experiences of this kind be evenly divided into phrases that are clearly and obviously alike, or phrases that are clearly and obviously different. Only after skill in this recognition is well

developed is it advisable to use songs in which the repetitions or differences are not so apparent. Older boys and girls who have not had previous experience of this kind need to start with songs in which the like and unlike phrases are easy to distinguish. However, these older pupils will usually sense longer phrase units (four and sometimes eight measures) as compared with shorter units which the younger children usually understand. The musical arrangement of songs with three phrases, five phrases, and phrases of uneven length will be easily recognized after the ear has been trained to notice repetitions and changes in melody and rhythm.

C. RHYTHMIC RESPONSE: LIKE AND UNLIKE PHRASES IN FAMILIAR SONGS AND IN INSTRUMENTAL MUSIC

Much of the music children hear on the piano and phonograph contains examples of identical or similar phrases which are easily recognized. Already the pupils are accustomed to demonstrating their feeling for successive musical phrases by rhythmic movements--a free circular movement of the arms, marching in different directions, and so on. See Chapter IV, p. 53, for more details.

As the pupils give closer attention to the exact melodic and rhythmic content of each phrase as it is heard, they begin to adjust these same activities to show their increasing comprehension of the form of the music. As the music of "Roundelay" is played, the class may respond to the first phrase of the music and to all like phrases with the circular arm movement. Perhaps they will simply listen quietly to the other phrases, or one group or row of pupils may respond to the repeated phrases and another group to the contrasting phrases.

Roundelay (Play a Tune, p. 46)

ROBERT SCHUMANN

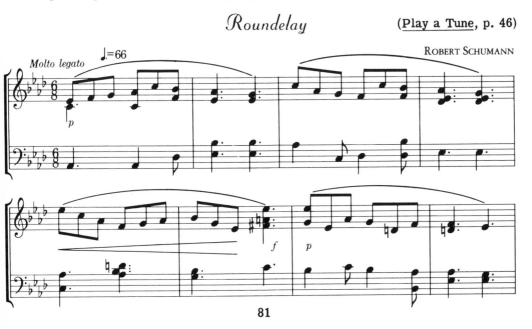

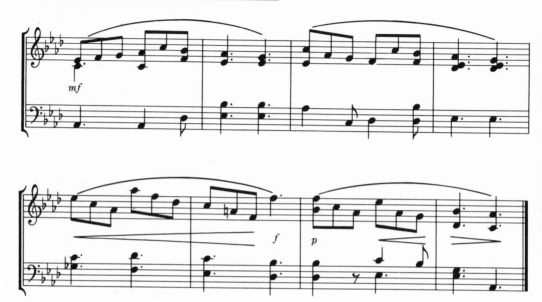

When a march such as "Tiptoe March" is being played, a member of the class or a group of children may respond by marching forward in the ordinary manner each time a repeated phrase is heard, but marking time in place, or marching on tiptoe, or making some different response when contrasting phrases are played. Many similar adaptations of the familiar phrasing activities may be used to show this recognition of like and unlike phrases.

Tiptoe March

(Play a Tune, p. 38)

ITALIAN FOLK TUNE

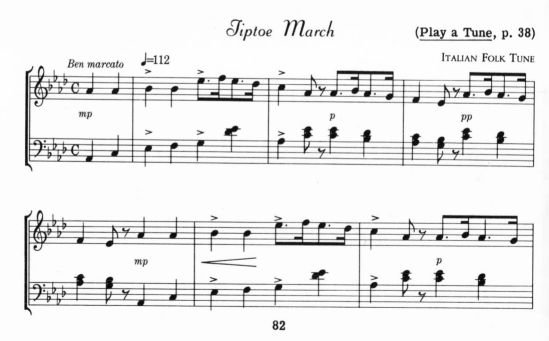

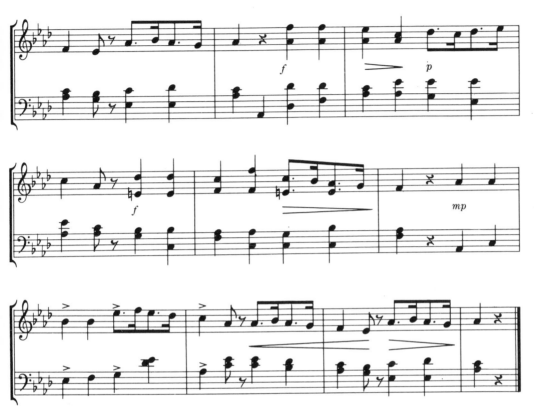

It is most important that the songs or instrumental selections for these activities be familiar through previous experiences in simple phrasing and rhythmic actions, or in singing or listening, in order that the children may easily recognize the phrases and have some understanding as to when to expect them to be repeated. It is not reasonable to think that children can make a good rhythmic response to anything as short as a musical phrase, with a feeling of muscular control and balance, if they are unfamiliar with the music. To get the real feeling of the entire sweep of a phrase, they must be ready to start the response at the very beginning.

For some of the activities suggested in other chapters of this book, the choice of music to be sung or played is limited to that which includes only certain kinds of measures or note values. There are no such limitations on the music which may be used for phrase recognition. Care should be taken, however, that the music is performed in such a way that the phrases are clearly and smoothly defined.

In addition to the selections included in this chapter, folk dances are usually very suitable for the experiences herein described because the short melodies permit much repetition of the phrases in a natural manner. Some of the folk dances included in Chapter I (pp. 18-20) can be used here as well.

The following selections from Play a Tune of The World of Music series will provide additional material for response to repeated phrases. A list follows:

I'll Tend My Sheep	p. 10	Chorale	p. 56
Gently My Johnny	p. 14	Theme, Symphony No. 5	p. 57
Song of the Shepherdess	p. 20	Minuet, Symphony in B♭	p. 58
Passepied	p. 25	Bacchanale	p. 58
Musette	p. 28	Minuet	p. 59
Waltz	p. 40	A Happy Story	p. 68
Rondo, Sonata No. 2	p. 53	Sweet Dreams	p. 70
Gavotte	p. 54	Slavonic Dance	p. 78

Other well-known selections suitable for these activities include

Klappdans	Swedish Folk Dance
Ace of Diamonds	Danish Folk Dance
Amaryllis	Ghys
Le Secret	Gautier
La Czarine	Ganne

Many of the selections listed are available on phonograph records. It is suggested that teachers who are interested in such recordings consult the educational catalogs or write the educational departments of the various record companies.

D. RESPONSE TO PHRASE REPETITION THROUGH RHYTHM INSTRUMENTS

The children have already become accustomed to the use of various groups of rhythm instruments to indicate their feeling for phrases in the music. (See Chapter IV, p. 54.) In carrying this experience further in connection with the activities described in this chapter, a familiar selection including a repeated phrase is played. One group of players, perhaps those with the rattle-jingle instruments, plays on the first phrase and every repetition of it, while all the other instruments play on all the contrasting phrases. When similar selections are played, the other groups or families of instruments each take a turn playing the repeated phrases. In case there is more than one phrase which is repeated, a certain group of instruments is chosen for each phrase, and plays only when this phrase and repetitions of it are heard. The same activity can be carried out as an accompaniment for songs which contain repeated phrases.

The Danish folk dance, "Ace of Diamonds," has three different musical phrases, A, B, and C, each of which is repeated. This music can be used with rhythm instruments to provide each of the three groups of instruments with its own special melody, and each group will play only where the special theme is heard. The music presented in this chapter and the other selections listed above are suitable also for use with groups of rhythm instruments.

Ace of Diamonds

DANISH FOLK DANCE

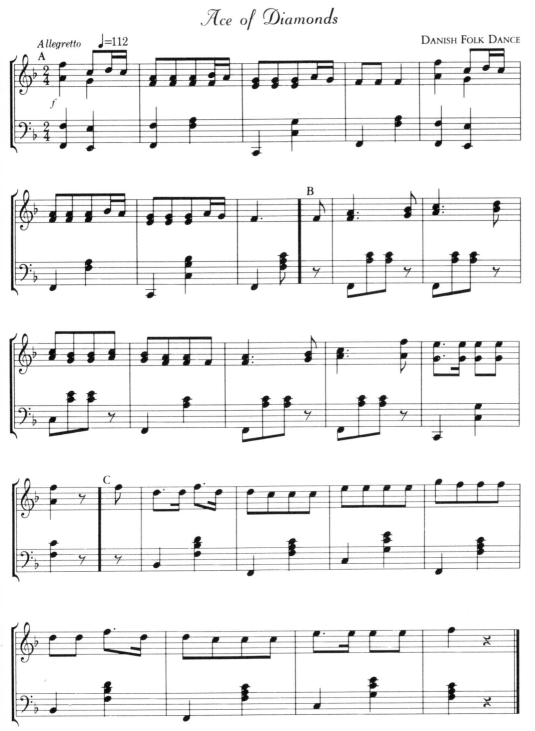

85

E. CREATIVE RESPONSE TO LIKE AND UNLIKE PHRASES

After a class has had some experience with these varied activities for responding to repeated and contrasted phrases, the children will enjoy making up phrase games of their own. They probably have noticed that in folk dances and games the steps or actions for recurring phrases in the music are either identical or very similar. This fact, along with the other experiences described in this chapter for making the rhythmic response change when the phrase changes, should suggest to the pupils that they will probably want to use the same steps or movements for phrase repetitions when creating original responses. The actual activity created is not important. The significant factor is that the children feel the need for making the same or a similar response for phrases that are alike, and a different response for contrasting phrases.

The resourceful teacher and a class accustomed to self-expression will enjoy devising many ways of showing their recognition of phrase repetition.

F. SIMULTANEOUS ACTIVITIES

The teacher should not wait to begin the activities presented in Chapter VIII and the succeeding chapters until all of the experiences in Chapter VII have been completed. Better results will be obtained if Chapter VII is carried on simultaneously with the steps that follow.

Chapter *VIII*
First Presentation of Rhythmic Notation

A. PREREQUISITE EXPERIENCE

Before beginning the activities described in the succeeding paragraphs, the children should have had abundant experience in responding rhythmically to music which includes the following kinds of notes and rhythmic patterns:

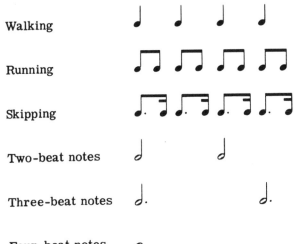

Walking

Running

Skipping

Two-beat notes

Three-beat notes

Four-beat notes

Pupils should be able to make prompt and accurate rhythmic response when they hear music in which any of the notes or rhythmic patterns given above clearly predominate. Unless they can recognize and respond to the music without making mistakes, when the selections on pages 71-78 are played, they are not yet prepared for the association of these rhythms with their notation.

The piano selections to which reference has been made include at least eight measures of each rhythmic pattern every time that pattern appears. The children are not asked to listen and respond to music in which the note values are changed so frequently that there is little or no time for adjustment to each change. All of these previous activities have been directed by the ear, <u>by listening to the music</u>, and each rhythmic pattern, whenever it appears, has predominated for a sufficient length of time to make recognition and response practical and easy.

If, under these circumstances, the children still are unable to make accurate rhythmic response in the activities listed in Chapters II, III, V, and VI, they are <u>not</u> ready to proceed with Chapter VIII. The physical feeling for the rhythm is all-important; without this feeling further progress will be slow and uncertain. The

87

experiences described in Chapter VII, however, can be conducted simultaneously with those in this chapter.

The contents of this chapter aim to present the notation symbols for the notes and rhythmic patterns that by this time are thoroughly familiar to the children through listening and movement, and to provide the varied activities necessary to give the children wide experience with these symbols as they appear in music.

B. PROCEDURE

(1) PRESENTATION OF NOTATION FOR WALKING, RUNNING, AND SKIPPING MUSIC

(a)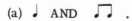

The rhythmic pattern for the melody of four phrases of a simple, familiar selection such as the "Theme" by Mozart, on page **33**, is written on the board or on a chart. Instead of the melody being in quarter notes throughout as it was originally written, however, the second and fourth phrases are written with ♫ for each ♩. As a result the four phrases appear like this:

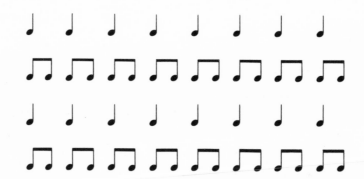

No measure bars have been included, and the final measure of each phrase has been made to include two quarter notes or four eighth notes in order to make the note content exactly the same as that of other measures. The class can, as a result, concentrate on the symbols for walking notes and running notes only. These notes must be written with note heads and stems large enough to be seen and recognized plainly from any place in the room. The phrases are numbered so that it will be possible to call attention to any one of them easily. The notes on the board or chart should be placed low enough to be within reach of the children.

The lesson may proceed as follows:

1. Teacher: "Boys and girls, please close your eyes and listen while I play. When I stop I want you to tell me what kind of music you have heard. Is it running, walking, or skipping?"

2. The teacher plays the first two phrases of the theme on page 33, Chapter II, with the note values changed to fit phrases 1 and 2 on page 35, with walking notes in the first phrase and running notes in the second, thus:

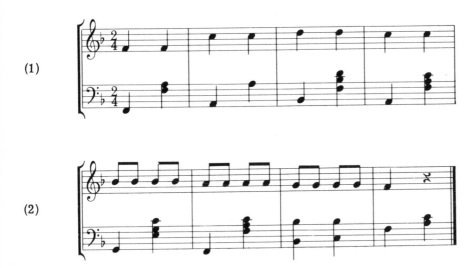

3. The pupils will probably answer, "We heard some walking notes and some running notes." Discussion should be permitted and it may be desirable to play these two phrases again.

4. Teacher: "Now while you look at the notes on the board (or chart) I'll play the music. I wonder if you can tell me which notes are the walking notes, and which are the running notes."

5. The teacher plays all four phrases of the music, alternating the note values as outlined. She indicates the beginning of each phrase by saying "second phrase" as she starts the second phrase, "third phrase" as she begins the third, and so on.

6. Teacher: "Who can show me which notes were the ones you saw when I played the walking music?" Some pupil points to the correct notes. The same procedure is used in identifying the contrasting running notes. There can be some discussion of the difference in appearance between the two kinds of notes, and it may be necessary to play the music once more in order to make the association of the <u>appearance</u> and <u>sound</u> clear in the minds of all the pupils.

7. The teacher next plays several short excerpts from compositions, in each of which either quarter notes or eighth notes predominate. The selections presented in Chapters II, III, and VI provide a variety of music for a wide experience of this kind. Any selections used for this activity must be in 2/4, 3/4, or 4/4 measure. It is important that the children always <u>listen first</u>, then indicate the kind of notes they hear by pointing to those on the board or chart, or by saying, "Walking notes like those in the first line," etc. This experience should continue until the association between the notes <u>heard</u> and the notes <u>seen</u> is almost automatic.

8. The teacher, pointing to the walking notes, asks, "Does anyone know another name for these walking notes?" If no one answers, the teacher tells the group that they are called <u>quarter</u> notes. Pupils should be informed that a quarter note sometimes looks like this: ♩ , and sometimes like this ♩ . It depends on the position on the staff; for example,

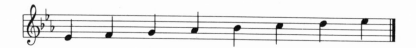

But regardless of the direction of its stem, it still remains a quarter note.

9. The same type of experience is provided for learning that another name for the running note is eighth note. Children will be interested to see the different representations that are possible with eighth notes. Two eighth notes together can be written in two ways: ♫ or ♪ ♪. When there are four of them they may be written ♪ ♪ ♪ ♪ or ♫♫ or ♪ ♪ ♫ As with quarter notes, sometimes the stems point down ♭ ♭ ♫ instead of up. It all depends on how high they come on the staff. In this early work the eighth notes always appear in groups of two or four. The reading of music with separate eighth notes presents some complicated rhythmic problems, and is an activity which should be deferred until some time later. No mention is made of the fractional or relative value of the eighth note and the quarter note. This experience is only concerned with the recognition of the appearance of the notes and their sound.

10. A class of children old enough to use <u>Rhythms and Rimes</u> (The World of Music series) or any similar book will be interested to learn that two or more running eighth notes in songs are usually written ♪ ♪ , while in instrumental music they appear like this: ♫ . They will soon discover for themselves through familiar songs that when eighth notes connected by a bar do appear in songs, there is only one word or syllable for notes so connected. When the eighth notes are written ♪ ♪ , each note has a separate word or syllable. For example, "Nine Red Horsemen" (<u>Rhythms and Rimes</u>, p. 144), "See What Grace" (<u>Songs of Many Lands</u>, p. 50), and "Colly, My Cow" (<u>Blending Voices</u>, p. 45), will provide illustrations of this.

Ample experience with these activities should be provided before continuing with the next section. It depends upon the maturity of the children; some classes can cover easily in one lesson most of the activities just described and be ready to proceed further. Others may need many days of such experience before their powers of correlating the ear, the eye, and bodily movement readily are developed. Drill activities to provide additional experience are suggested under paragraph 3 on page 92.

(b) ♩. ♪ AND ♫

During the same lesson or in a following one the teacher places on the board or a chart a succession of four or five groups of the rhythmic pattern ♩. ♪ . Successions of quarter notes and eighth notes are also presented for comparison. Then the teacher plays "Turkey in the Straw," p. 27, or "Rig-a-jig," p. 38, or any other selection in 2/4, 3/4, or 4/4 measure in which the predominant rhythmic figure in the melody is ♩. ♪ . The same plan as was used for introducing the notation ♩ and ♫ is followed here; the children first listen to the music and discover that it suggests skipping. Then when they look at the notes on the board they can easily recognize ♩. ♪ as the skipping pattern.

As was the case with running notes, the skipping notes always appear in pairs or in fours. Two together are generally written ♪. ♪ in songs, and ♪. ♪ in instrumental music; four are frequently written ♪. ♪♪. ♪ in songs, and ♪.♪♪.♪ or ♪.♪♪.♪ in instrumental compositions, although the latter notations are also used in vocal music when there are two or four notes to be sung to one syllable in the text of the song. Like walking and running notes, the stems may point downward or upward, according to their location on the staff.

The children should learn the names of the notes in this skipping combination: dotted eighth note and sixteenth note. It is recommended that for the present teachers and classes continue to refer to all of the notes presented in this section as "skipping," "running," or "walking" notes or music, the pupils learning the new terminology gradually.

The question may be raised: why not introduce ♩ ♪♩ ♪ and ♪₇♩ ♪₇♩ in 6/8 measure as "skipping music" at this point? It is true that these also are rhythmic patterns for music which suggests skipping. But they are deferred until a later time and a later chapter, as are other "skipping" or long-short combinations such as ♩. ♪♩. ♪ in 2/2 and 4/2 measure, and ♪.♪ ♪ ♪ in 3/8 or 4/8 measure. For the present the pupils are introduced only to the manner in which the rhythms with which they are familiar are notated when the <u>quarter note</u> is the beat unit or "walking" note. Too rapid introduction of music in which notes other than the quarter notes are used as the beat unit has proved to be confusing to many children. The quarter note is the fundamental beat note, and a large proportion of the world's music, especially the music which children will play and sing, is written with the quarter note as the unit of measurement. However, every class should have abundant experience in higher grades with music in which other notes are employed as beat units.

(2) PRESENTATION OF NOTATION OF TWO-BEAT, THREE-BEAT, AND FOUR-BEAT NOTES

When the children are able to recognize "walking," "running," and "skipping" notes when they <u>see</u> them as well as when they <u>hear</u> them, they are ready to be introduced to the notation of two-beat, three-beat, and four-beat notes. The note successions found in the melody line of "Improvisation 1," p. 66, are written on the board, thus:

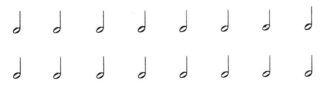

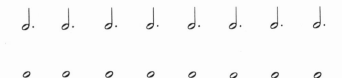

While the class listens, using their arms to mark the beats (as in Chapter V, p. 61), the first eight measures of "Improvisation 1" are played. The music stops and the class recognizes the notes they have heard as two-beat notes. Following the same procedure as was used for the introduction of ♩ and ♫ , the class now watches the successions of ♩ , ♩. , and ○ on the board while the entire "Improvisation 1" is played. As the children swing their arms to mark the beats and watch the notes, they discover the difference between the two-beat, the three-beat, and the four-beat notes. If the teacher can have someone point to each phrase as it is played, recognition of these notes by every member of the class will be more rapid. When the music stops, the relative values of the three new notes are pointed out by the children and discussed. The names "half note," "dotted half note," and "whole note" are presented, as well as details about the writing of the notes, in the same way as was done with the walking, running, and skipping notes. No mathematical study of the function of the dot after the half note is made. Through rhythmic activity and sight the children recognize ♩ as a two-beat note and ♩. as a three-beat note, and will naturally assume that the dot is responsible for the extra beat. No further understanding is necessary at this time if steady rhythmic response is made to the notes.

(3) PRACTICE GAMES FOR AURAL AND VISUAL RECOGNITION OF RHYTHMIC PATTERNS

As soon as the children are familiar with the notation of two or more rhythmic patterns, the following activities are suggested to establish the association between rhythms and their notation.

(a) ASSOCIATING NOTES HEARD WITH THOSE SEEN

Music is played and the children listen and then choose the correct notation from the groups of notes on the board or on flash cards to fit what is heard. For example, if the teacher plays "Turkish March," p. 59, the children should select the group of notes on the board or flash card containing the pattern ♩ ♩ ♩ ♩ |

♩ ♩ ♩ ♩   or   ♩ ♩ | ○ |

The teacher may sing, using a neutral syllable (loo or tah), the following verse of "Yankee Doodle:"

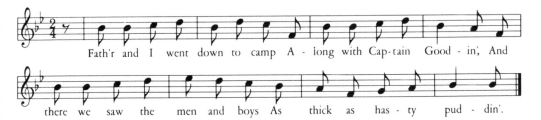

This illustrates a certain rhythmic pattern. The children listen, recognize the notes as running notes and, since this is a song, they choose the flash card with ♪♪♪♪ | ♪♪♪♪ . Music containing other familiar rhythmic patterns may be played or sung while the children identify the predominating pattern heard in each selection. Rhythm instruments are also very helpful for producing groups of notes for recognition.

(b) NAMING THE NOTES SEEN AND HEARD

The children name the kinds of notes being played as they point to them: "quarter notes," "half notes," "eighth notes," etc.

(c) RESPONDING TO THE NOTES SEEN

As the teacher points to the notation of one of the familiar rhythmic patterns, the children demonstrate it rhythmically. For example, as she points to ♪. ♪♪ ♪ or ♫. ♫. , the child who is responding skips, or plays a skipping rhythm on a rhythm instrument; when the teacher's hand moves to ♩ , the child walks or plays a walking rhythm. When the teacher indicates ○ , the child changes to a four-beat response or plays a drum or gong with strike, swing, swing, swing. (See page 70). The teacher is not to change from ♪♪♪♪ or ♪. ♪♪. ♪ to ♩ ♩ , ♩. ♩. or ○ ○ , but always to proceed from ♩ ♩ ♩ ♩ to ♩ ♩ , ♩. ♩. or ○ ○ , since the quarter notes are the beat notes and set the tempo better for the longer notes, making the transition from one rhythm to another much smoother. It is perfectly satisfactory, however, to change from notes longer than quarter notes to ♪♪♪♪ and ♫. ♫. without the interpolation of ♩ ♩ ♩ ♩ .

Children, as they become familiar with the notes, will enjoy having certain members of the class point to groups of notes to which other pupils are to respond. This activity can be worked out sometimes in the form of a rhythmic "spelldown," allowing each child to continue as long as he makes accurate response. When he misses he goes to the end of the line.

LEARNING MUSIC THROUGH RHYTHM

It is essential in all experiences of this type that a strong feeling for steady beats be constantly maintained. It is also essential that each of the examples of various rhythmic patterns be long enough to allow the child to establish a smooth response to the rhythm before being asked to change. As an illustration, it requires at least four groups of skipping notes, ♫. ♫. ♫. ♫ to allow opportunity for establishing a smooth skipping movement; if a change is made too soon the child's feeling for an underlying rhythmic pulsation may be lost.

The children who remain at their seats should always participate, using their hands and arms for rhythmic movement and following the notes as the person at the board or with the flash cards indicates them. Sometimes they can softly and lightly scan the rhythmic patterns, repeating the same neutral syllable, such as tah, for each note, making it long or short so as to fit the pattern. Illustrations show the following results:

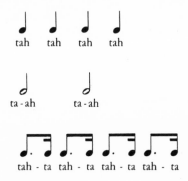

If done very lightly this scanning can prove to be a very significant intermediate step, linking the skill and understanding acquired through rhythmic movement directly with its application to vocal reading of songs. This is particularly feasible as an activity for older children.

(4) WRITING THE NOTATION OF FAMILIAR RHYTHMIC PATTERNS

It is important that children who are experienced and old enough to write notes easily learn to write these familiar rhythmic patterns. Some time should be taken to teach them how to make the various notes. For example:

- ○ = ○   (whole note)
- ○ with the addition of a stem   (|) = ♩   (half note)
- ○ with the addition of a stem (|) and a dot (.) = ♩.   (dotted half note)

In simplified form it may be expressed thus:

o = o (whole note)

o + | = ♩ (half note)

o + | + . = ♩. (dotted half note)

Quarter notes should not be written by filling in half notes. One quick line with the lengthwise side of a short piece of chalk will make a quarter note on the board without any difficulty. The following routine is suggested:

♩ + | = ♩ (quarter note)

♩ + | + ╲ (flag) = ♪ (eighth note)

♩ + | + ♩ + | + ‾ = ♫ (two eighth notes)

(5) CLASS PARTICIPATION IN THE LEARNING OF ROTE SONGS

From this point the children should be led to note these various rhythmic patterns whenever they appear in the notation of the familiar rote songs which they sing, having their books in their hands. The class can develop surprisingly in consciousness of rhythmic notation if a little attention is given from time to time to the notes in these familiar songs.

Many teachers, beginning with Grade II, teach some of the songs by rote with the books in the hands of the children. At any grade level where this is done the pupils will enjoy helping the teacher with a new rote song by looking at the music and telling her whether to make the words of the first line walk or run or skip. For instance, in introducing such a song as "Peter Day" the children, looking at the notes and words, will be able to suggest that the word "Peter" in the first line and "Anna" in the third must <u>run</u> because the notes do, while most of the other notes <u>walk</u>. Children will usually find the two-beat notes for "Joe" and "go" also, and then will be interested to hear the teacher sing the song as they have suggested.

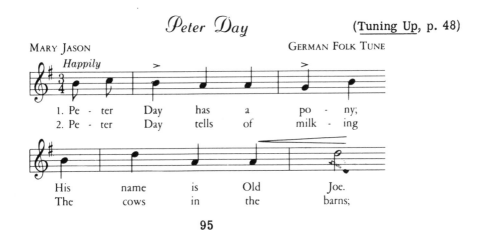

Peter Day   (Tuning Up, p. 48)

MARY JASON   GERMAN FOLK TUNE

1. Pe - ter Day has a po - ny;
2. Pe - ter Day tells of milk - ing

His name is Old Joe.
The cows in the barns;

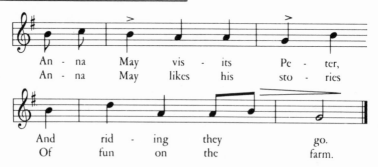

An - na May vis - its Pe - ter,
An - na May likes his sto - ries

And rid - ing they go.
Of fun on the farm.

Rote songs which include these familiar rhythmic patterns are to be found in any song books which the children may have at any grade level. They can be used to advantage to develop and improve attention to and understanding of the association between the rhythmic scheme of the words and that of the notes.

When the children are giving attention to the notation, songs in 6/8 measure are not recommended for use as yet, since they include a new, unfamiliar problem — the "walking" note in 6/8 measure is the dotted quarter note ($\downarrow$.) . Songs in 6/8 measure, therefore, will be used for rote singing, with no attention being given by the class to the notation.

Children also enjoy being questioned by the teacher as to whether or not she is singing a new song in correct rhythm. For example, when presenting a new song such as "The Christmas Tree," she may say, "I am going to sing the first phrase of this new song. Will you watch the notes and tell me if I am singing it just as it looks in your book?"

The Christmas Tree

(Tuning Up, p. 91)

FREDERICK H. MARTENS   HUNGARIAN FOLK TUNE

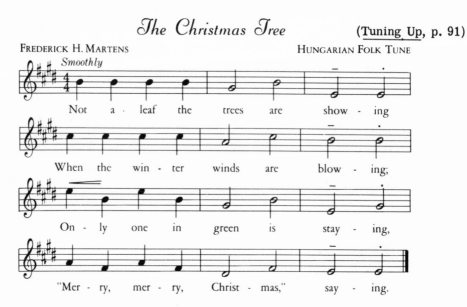

Not a leaf the trees are show - ing

When the win - ter winds are blow - ing;

On - ly one in green is stay - ing,

"Mer - ry, mer - ry, Christ - mas," say - ing.

96

After setting the tempo, the teacher sings the first phrase, as follows:

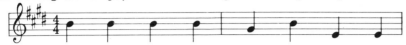

The alert child will be delighted to discover that the teacher sang all quarter notes, and that there are some two-beat notes in the phrase. The teacher may then ask some child to sing the phrase correctly. Having heard the melody sung, the child is concerned only with the reading of the correct rhythm. This device is valuable in developing notation-consciousness, since in their song books the children are inclined to watch words rather than notes.

(6) UNDERSTANDING OF RESTS

It is impossible to give very much attention to rhythmic notation of songs without encountering rests. Children are immediately curious about them, and will make their acquaintance easily and naturally if they are already familiar with the note equivalents of the rests. When the teacher introduces such a song as "If I Had a Doggie,"

If I Had a Doggie

(Tuning Up, p. 29)

KATHLEEN MALONE   FINNISH FOLK TUNE

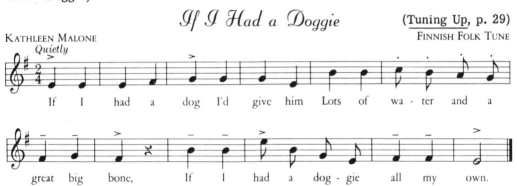

the children, in looking at the notes and words, will find the places where the music walks and where it runs. They will find the single two-beat note, and they will also notice the new sign or symbol at the end of the second phrase. They listen while the teacher sings the song. Sometimes she has to repeat it before they discover what happens after the word "bone." It may help to make them conscious of it if the teacher makes four downward arm swings as she sings "great big bone." They discover that there is one silent beat at the end of the phrase and learn to know that the sign is equal to a walking note, but silent. Thereafter they will always recognize and respond to the quarter rest when it appears, making it the signal for a very soft walking step when on the floor, or swinging the arm for it as for a quarter note when at their seats. It is an important part of the music; it must always be included, even though it indicates silence.

LEARNING MUSIC THROUGH RHYTHM

The half rest can easily be introduced through a song such as

The Snowman

(Tuning Up, p. 82)

MARY SMITH

YUGOSLAVIAN FOLK TUNE

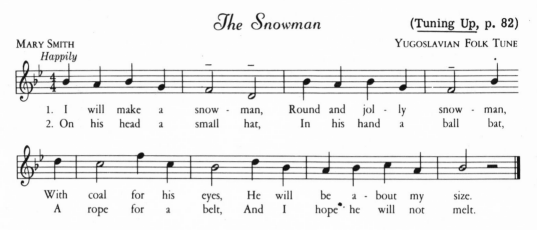

1. I will make a snow - man, Round and jol - ly snow - man,
2. On his head a small hat, In his hand a ball bat,

With coal for his eyes, He will be a - bout my size.
A rope for a belt, And I hope he will not melt.

If the children hear the two stanzas of the song, they will discover that the rest furnishes two beats of silence between the stanzas.

Later the class will also be interested in making the acquaintance of the eighth rest as it appears in

Travel

(Tuning Up, p. 80)

HOPE ANN RHODES

SPANISH FOLK TUNE

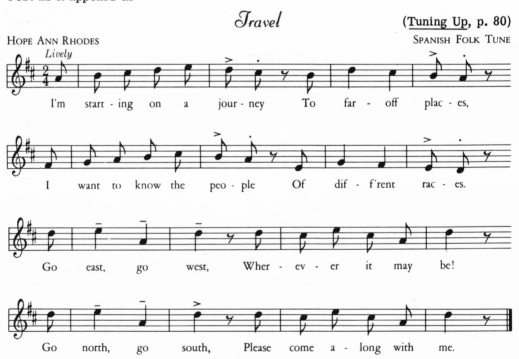

I'm start - ing on a jour - ney To far - off plac - es,

I want to know the peo - ple Of dif - f'rent rac - es.

Go east, go west, Wher - ev - er it may be!

Go north, go south, Please come a - long with me.

Since the eighth rest in most songs is very quickly slipped in, little attention need be given to developing any kind of response to it.

Songs for use in introducing these rests will be found in song books for all age levels.

(7) A GAME: WHERE DID THE MUSIC STOP?

An instrumental melody, or the music of a rote song including only familiar rhythmic patterns in 2/4, 3/4, or 4/4 measure, is written on the board. The teacher plays the melody or sings it with a neutral syllable, stopping on some note before the selection or song is completed. The children are to follow the melody and be ready to show which note was the last one heard. For example, the following melody can be used for such a game:

Themes from Amaryllis

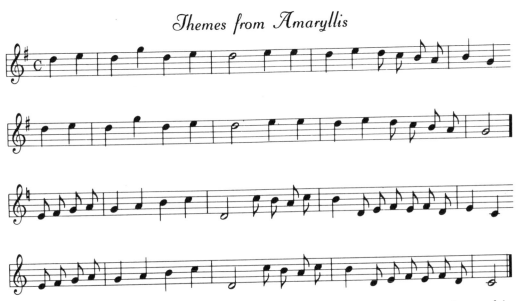

The melody only of the following selections from <u>Play a Tune</u> may be used in the same way:

Écossaise	p. 30
Rondo	p. 30
Bourrée	p. 32
March	p. 34
Cornelius March	p. 37

<u>Play a Tune</u> also includes many other compositions in 2/4, 3/4, and 4/4 measure in which the melody line is made up of the rhythmic patterns which are already familiar to the children.

The same game may be played by using the children's song books, if they learn to watch the <u>notes</u> and not the words. This method of teaching a rote song is also very interesting to children who have had enough experience to read the words and follow the notes as well. After several opportunities to play the game of telling (or showing) on which note the music stopped, they have usually heard the song a sufficient number of times to be ready to sing it with little or no help.

Chapter IX
Response to Accents in Music

Before the activities of this chapter are begun, it is important that the children have a wide variety of experiences in responding to the rhythmic swing of the music, and also in feeling and responding to the successive beats in the music, as outlined in the preceding chapters. The activities described in this chapter aim to lead the children to discover that some beats in music are stronger than others, and that each measure includes one strong beat and one or more weak beats. This is a most important step in the musical development of each member of the class: it is essential to all future rhythmic progress.

A. CHOICE OF MUSIC

The music for these different experiences can be furnished by singing songs, by playing the piano, by phonograph records, or by rhythmic patterns played on a rhythm instrument. However, since many of the responses require such active movement as to make singing a rather undesirable musical background, it is probable that in a large part of the experiences instrumental music will be used for accompaniment. When songs are used, a group selected from the whole class (or the teacher) should provide the music while the others respond.

Many selections which can be effectively used with these activities are included in this chapter. For some of the activities described in other chapters the choice of music to be sung or played is limited to that which includes only certain kinds of measures or note values. There are no such limitations here. Music in all kinds of measure and with all kinds of note values may be used for the experiences which follow. The only exception is marching, which requires music in duple or quadruple measure.

Each selection and song should have a very definite, clear, natural accent which says either "One, two," or "One, two, three," or "One, two, three, four." The "one" beat should be played with a stronger accent than the other beats, although care should be taken not to spoil the musical beauty through overemphasis. For the first activities suggested here, each selection must be confined to one kind of measure. It must not include a change of measure.

In addition to the music presented in this chapter, the following selections from Play a Tune are recommended as types of music which are satisfactory for these experiences:

LEARNING MUSIC THROUGH RHYTHM

(1) DUPLE MEASURE

Distinct "strong, weak" beat:

Écossaise No. 3	Schubert	p. 30
Flower Parade	Italian	p. 36
Russian Dance	Napravnik	p. 37
Song of the Gypsy	Hungarian	p. 62
Gavotte	Gillet	p. 27
Harlequin Columbine	Kleinmichel	p. 24

(2) TRIPLE MEASURE

Distinct "strong, weak, weak" beat:

Waltz	Schubert	p. 40
Waltz	Brahms	p. 40
Waltz, Opus 90, No. 14	Schubert	p. 48
Papillons	Schumann	p. 60
Minuet	Mozart	p. 47
Minuet	Haydn	p. 58
A Happy Story	German	p. 68
On the Village Green	Czech	p. 61

(3) QUADRUPLE MEASURE

Distinct "strong, weak, weak, weak" beat:

Passepied	Delibes	p. 25
Folk Dance	Danish	p. 25
Theme-Sonata, Opus 14, No. 2	Beethoven	p. 27
March	Gounod	p. 31
March from Lenore Symphony	Raff	p. 32
Song without Words	Mendelssohn	p. 34
Christmas Tree March	Gade	p. 35
Cavalry March	Finnish	p. 36

B. PROCEDURE

There are many different ways to develop recognition of and response to the accent in music. The teacher can choose from the suggestions offered those which seem most suitable to her group and to the immediate situation. The general sequence in which they may be introduced most easily is listed in the following order.

(1) PENDULUM SWING

The children stand and swing arms, both arms together, from side to side, pendulum fashion, to music such as the following:

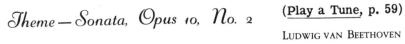

Theme — Sonata, Opus 10, No. 2 (Play a Tune, p. 59)

LUDWIG VAN BEETHOVEN

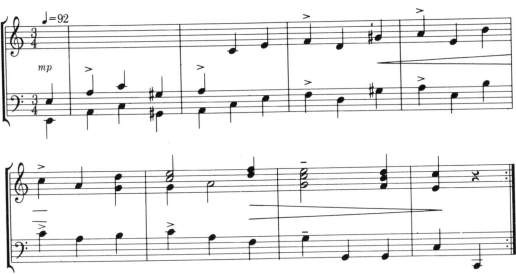

On the strong beats both arms will be swung vigorously and high, and parallel to the floor. For each weaker beat the arms will not swing high but rather in an easy, lazy movement. The children will learn in the course of time that in these experiences it is best for all to start together, with arms swinging from the same side and in the same rhythmic movement. If they begin by simply swinging in response to the beats in the music, without accent, they gradually will feel and begin to show the accented beats. This is another activity which should sometimes be carried on with eyes closed in order to avoid watching what the others are doing and to prevent interference with individual reaction.

(2) ARM MOVEMENTS

When space for swinging the arms freely is not available, the children may indicate their feeling for the accent by pushing both hands downward on the strong beats and bringing them upward on each weak beat. For example, triple measure would be demonstrated in this way:

(a) Down—a movement so vigorous that the hands rebound almost to original position
(b) Up lightly—second beat
(c) Up still more lightly—third beat
(d) Down again vigorously—first beat of the new measure, etc.

Both of the preceding activities are inaudible ones. It is very important that the class master one or both of these methods of silent response to accented and unaccented beats, because an audible response cannot be used in connection with many of the activities which follow. For additional experience, however, some audible responses in these experiences are now offered.

(3) STRONG, WEAK, ETC.

The class listens to music in duple measure such as the following:

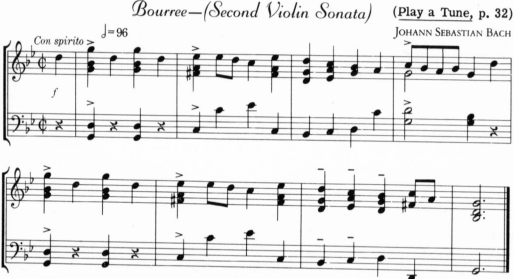

Bourree—(Second Violin Sonata) (Play a Tune, p. 32)

JOHANN SEBASTIAN BACH

The children indicate the accented and unaccented beats in the music by one of the responses already suggested in paragraphs 1 and 2. As they make their movement, they give further emphasis to their response by saying aloud the word "strong" with every heavy, accented beat, and the word "weak" with the light, unaccented beats. They soon discover that the music moves along with a "strong, weak" pattern. Many classes will gain in skill and understanding more rapidly if they concentrate on the accented beat at first, until they sense it quickly. Then they will be making a "down, up" movement and saying "strong" with each accented downward movement. If they feel these strong beats easily they will soon accurately fit the correct number of weak beats into the light movements they are making between the accents.

This should also be carried on through the use of familiar songs having clearly defined measure. Part of the class (or the teacher) may sing the song, preferably with a neutral syllable, while the rest of the group respond with movements, saying "strong, weak", etc.

In the same way the children listen to music in triple measure, such as

Playing in the Sun (Rhythms and Rimes, p. 133)

LOUISE AYRES GARNETT

FRENCH FOLK TUNE

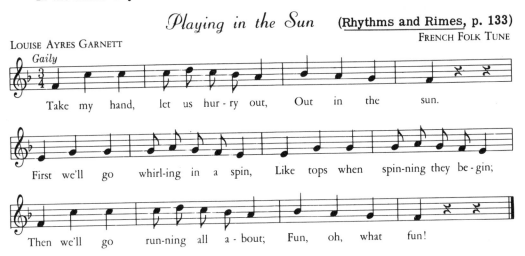

Take my hand, let us hur-ry out, Out in the sun.

First we'll go whirl-ing in a spin, Like tops when spin-ning they be-gin;

Then we'll go run-ning all a-bout; Fun, oh, what fun!

Through accented and unaccented movements they discover that the melody says, "strong, weak, weak," etc. and they say these words aloud as they make rhythmic response. Also, after listening and responding to a song or selection in quadruple measure, such as the one which follows, they find themselves saying, "strong, weak, weak, weak," etc.

Allegro—Sonata No. 5 (Play a Tune, p. 46)

FRANZ JOSEPH HAYDN

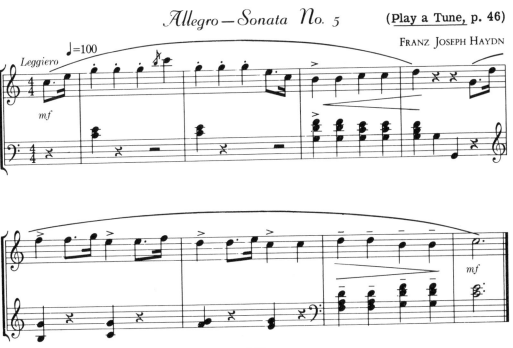

105

Thus, through listening to and rhythmic movement with these and a variety of other selections and songs in duple, triple, and quadruple measure, the children discover these three kinds of musical patterns of accented and unaccented beats. Music used for this purpose must be well accented; it must plainly reveal the measure or the children will have difficulty in making their own discoveries.

To make sure that opportunity is given in these responses for individual development, it is best sometimes for the children to say the words, "strong" and "weak" silently to themselves during the first few measures, and to raise their hands when they are sure which of the three possible combinations they hear. When several have raised their hands, they can compare their discoveries and decide on the correct combination of accented and unaccented beats. For variety, at other times they will simply say aloud "strong, weak," etc., as soon as they discover the kind of music they are hearing. Care must be taken that all these speaking responses are made lightly. "Strong" should not be boisterous, and "weak" should be spoken very softly.

(4) "ONE, TWO," ETC.

The children listen and move in the same way as was suggested under 3, but instead of saying, "Strong, weak," etc., they count "One, two," or "One, two, three," or "One, two, three, four," according to the measure of the music. Also it is suggested that they be allowed to concentrate first on developing a strong feeling for the "one." If "one" can be recognized and a response be always made to it there will be no difficulty in finding the number of beats coming between the "ones." If the children become confused from time to time with new music, they should learn always to stop and find the "ones" throughout the movement, and then find the other beats. Additional activities of this kind are to be found in Music Activities and Practices in the Kindergarten and Elementary Grades, by Mabelle Glenn, p. 44 (or in Music Teaching in the Kindergarten and Primary Grades, by Mabelle Glenn, p. 66).

(5) MARCHING

With music in duple and quadruple measures, the children march with a heavy step on the strong beats and a very soft, light step on the weaker beats. It can be suggested to them that their marching steps be very light until they feel a strong beat. Then they are to make their feet follow the music, marching on strong and weak beats as the music tells them to do. "Marche Militaire" is an excellent composition for the first experience with this activity.

Marche Militaire

FRANZ SCHUBERT

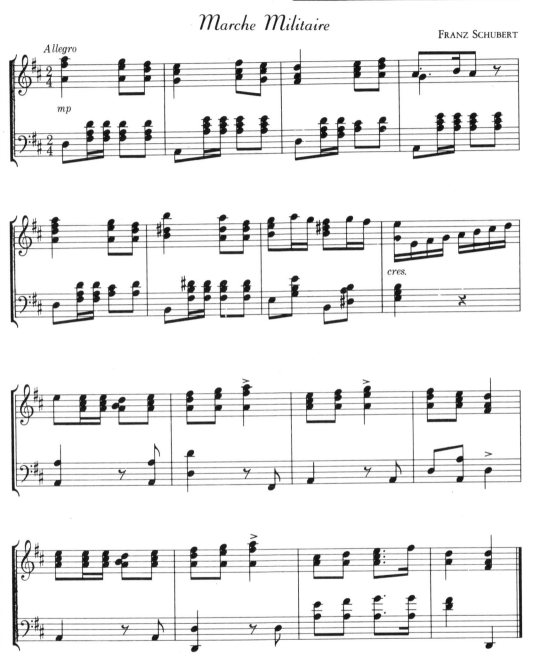

The teacher should emphasize the importance of always using the <u>left</u> foot on the accent when marching. Music in triple measure should not be used for this activity since the heavy step will alternate from the right foot to the left foot, and thus confuse the children.

(6) CLAPPING

The children listen to instrumental music or to a rhythmic song and clap softly to the music. As soon as they discover the pattern of accents and weaker beats in the music, they begin to indicate this through strong and weak clapping. Some groups have found that if the fingertips are used on weak beats, and a light hand clap on the strong beats, the activity shows contrast without becoming noisy.

C. DRAMATIZATION OF SONGS

While the children are learning to recognize and respond to accented and un-accented beats, in music, action songs which emphasize these accents through movements which interpret the words are very valuable. Many songs are to be found in the pupils' books of the various music series in general use which lend themselves admirably to these experiences. One song may suggest bouncing a ball; another may offer opportunity for rowing a boat; others may suggest the swinging of a pendulum, ringing of a church bell, playing a hand organ, a blacksmith pounding on his anvil, swinging a sickle, scrubbing and ironing clothes, and many other such activities. The songs used should have been well learned before any action is attempted. Teachers often will be agreeably surprised at suggestions children themselves will offer; suitable suggestions should be tried out frequently. Excellent suggestions for such song dramatization for older boys and girls will be found in Dramatized Ballads by Tobitt and White (E. P. Dutton and Company).

D. RHYTHM INSTRUMENTS

The children have already had experience in playing rhythm instruments to show the contrasting rhythms they hear in music (p. 41). They must now develop further discrimination by indicating with their instruments the accented and un-accented beats they hear in songs or instrumental selections. One group of instruments is chosen to play on the strong beats only, while the others play very softly on the weak beats. Each group has its turn at playing on the accented beats, while the others come in on the light beats. The children soon begin to become conscious of tone-color contrasts among the instruments, and of various degrees of volume and intensity. Before long they begin to feel the lack of balance that occurs when the heavier percussion instruments play, even lightly, on unaccented beats. They also discover that some instruments, namely the large hand drum or tom tom, can produce sounds with a wide variation in volume and intensity, and thus can be played so as to indicate both accented and unaccented beats clearly. In this way a definite vocabulary of orchestral effects and combinations of instruments is built up to help the children in later creative orchestration.

E. VISUAL REPRESENTATION OF MEASURE

As the children listen to songs or instrumental selections they indicate the accented or unaccented beats on the board with long and short marks like these:

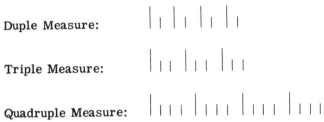

This provides valuable experience through a new and interesting movement activity, and the children enjoy it. However, the teacher is cautioned against carrying such devices past their point of usefulness through overemphasis, or through the type of distortion which has the children struggling so hard to make complicated, rhythmic drawings that they lose all feeling for the music.

F. RESPONSE TO CHANGES IN MEASURE

After the class has had wide experience in sensing and responding to the meter of songs and selections each of which is confined to one kind of measure, they will enjoy carrying on the same activities while they listen to music in which the measure changes. The selections which follow can be used separately for the activities suggested earlier in the chapter. If, however, the first three of these selections are played without pause, they provide an interesting sequence of measure changes. Care should be taken in playing this music that the tempo of the beat is changed very little or not at all when the measure in the music changes. Note that a tempo marking is given for the first selection on page 110. The two compositions which follow should be played at the same rate of speed. In changing from one kind of measure to another, there must be no break or halt in the music to reveal the change to the class; they should sense the change from the order of the strong and weak beats in the music.

Only silent methods of swinging and beating should be used here. If audible responses are used, the children will be unable to hear the change in measure when it occurs in the music. The children will find that they can feel the change and respond much more easily and quickly if their eyes are closed.

Moment Musical

(Play a Tune, p. 59)

FRANZ SCHUBERT
Opus 24

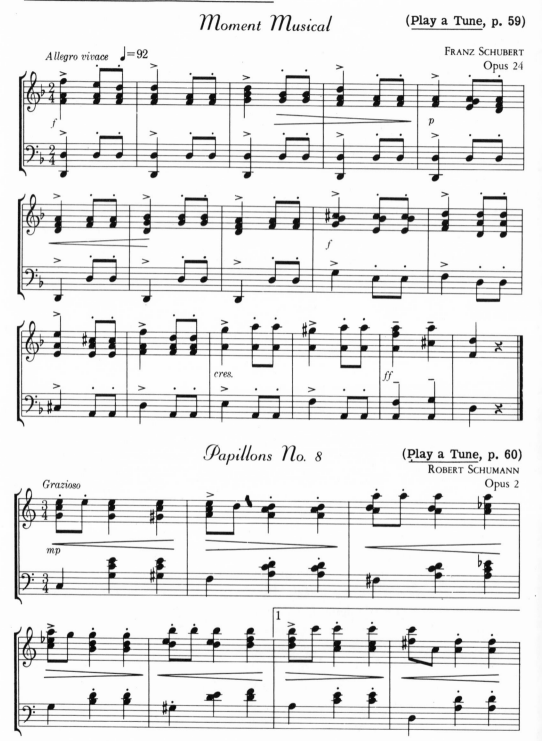

Papillons No. 8

(Play a Tune, p. 60)

ROBERT SCHUMANN
Opus 2

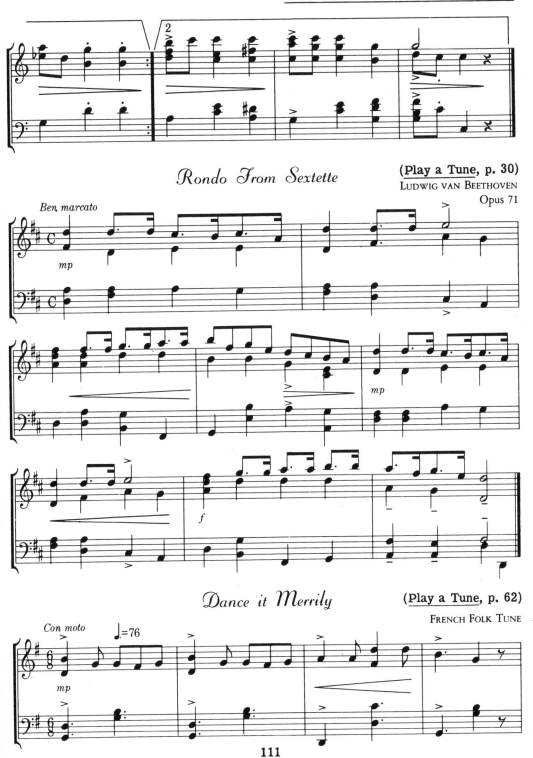

Rondo From Sextette

(Play a Tune, p. 30)
Ludwig van Beethoven
Opus 71

Dance it Merrily

(Play a Tune, p. 62)
French Folk Tune

111

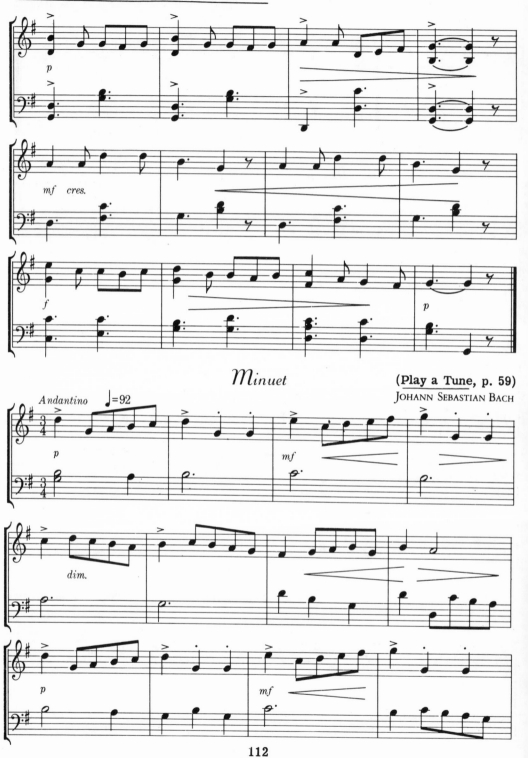

Minuet

(Play a Tune, p. 59)

JOHANN SEBASTIAN BACH

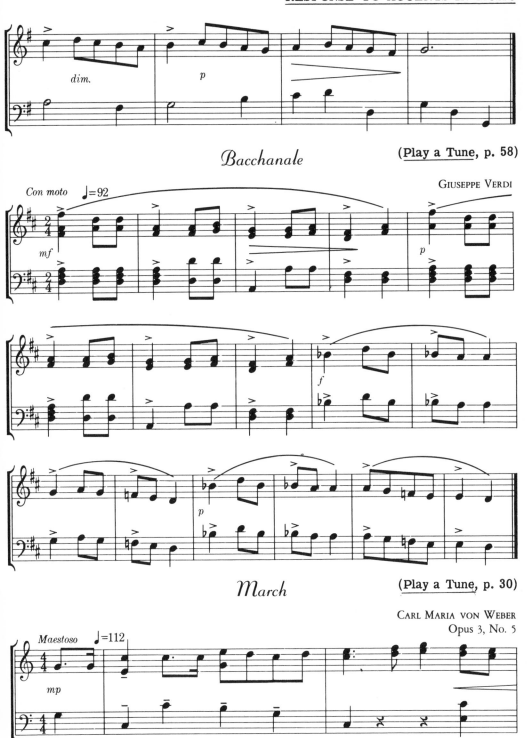

Bacchanale (Play a Tune, p. 58)

GIUSEPPE VERDI

March (Play a Tune, p. 30)

CARL MARIA VON WEBER
Opus 3, No. 5

113

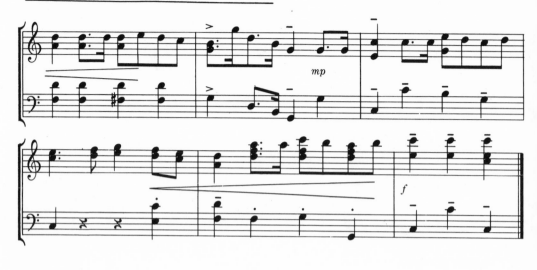

Minuet

(Play a Tune, p. 47)

WOLFGANG AMADEUS MOZART

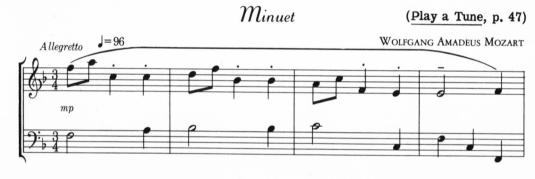

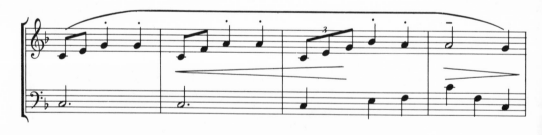

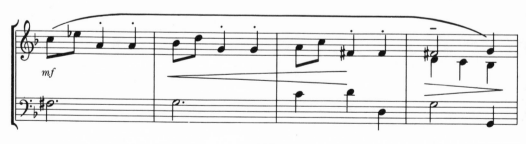

114

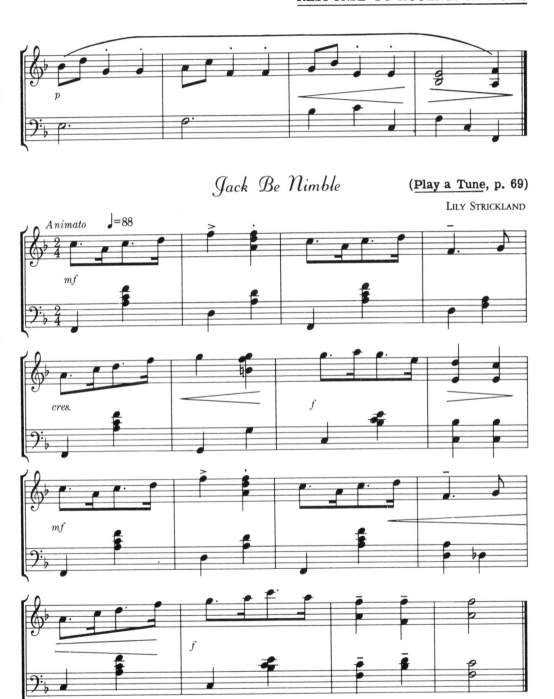

Jack Be Nimble
(Play a Tune, p. 69)

LILY STRICKLAND

Chapter X
The Measure Bar
and the Measure Signature

The activities described in this chapter are designed to follow considerable experience along the lines suggested in Chapter IX. The children should be able to recognize and respond to the strong and weak beats in music before continuing with the work presented on the following pages.

It is possible that some of the familiar songs suggested may have previously been taught by rote, while others may have been read by the class for the understanding of note values, but with no definite attention being directed to measure signatures and bar lines.

A. DISCOVERY OF THE FUNCTION OF THE MEASURE BAR

(1) QUADRUPLE MEASURE

With books open, the children sing a familiar song in quadruple measure in which the quarter note receives one beat. Either of the following is a good example.

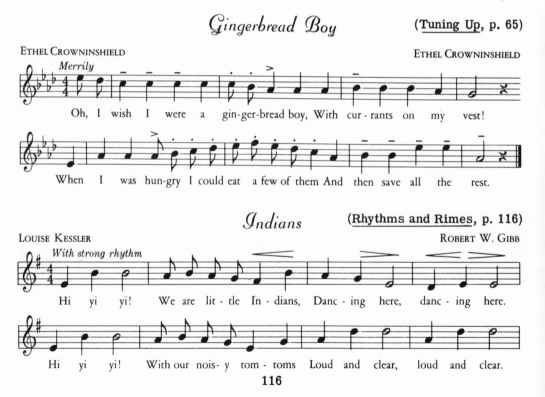

Gingerbread Boy
(Tuning Up, p. 65)

ETHEL CROWNINSHIELD

ETHEL CROWNINSHIELD

Merrily

Oh, I wish I were a gin-ger-bread boy, With cur-rants on my vest!

When I was hun-gry I could eat a few of them And then save all the rest.

Indians
(Rhythms and Rimes, p. 116)

LOUISE KESSLER

ROBERT W. GIBB

With strong rhythm

Hi yi yi! We are lit-tle In-dians, Danc-ing here, danc-ing here.

Hi yi yi! With our nois-y tom-toms Loud and clear, loud and clear.

116

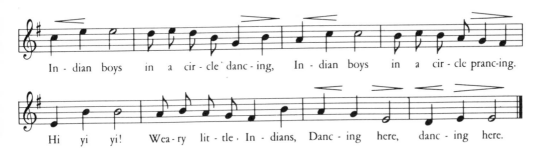

In - dian boys in a cir - cle danc - ing, In - dian boys in a cir - cle pranc-ing.

Hi yi yi! Wea - ry lit - tle In - dians, Danc - ing here, danc - ing here.

The strong beats are definitely accented in the singing and the children show the accented and unaccented beats by moving their hands as they sing. They discover which words in each phrase are sung on the strong beats. They are then led to notice the vertical line which appears before the strongly accented notes or "ones" in the music. In the event that no one knows what these lines are called the teacher identifies the line as a <u>measure</u> bar.

In the song "Indians" the children discover that no measure bar is placed before a "one" beat appearing at the beginning of a new line or staff of music. The music between the measure bars is now called by its rightful name--a measure of music.

(2) TRIPLE MEASURE

A familiar song in triple measure is sung from the books, such as

The Street Organ

(Tuning Up, p. 95)

MARY JASON

YUGOSLAVIAN FOLK TUNE

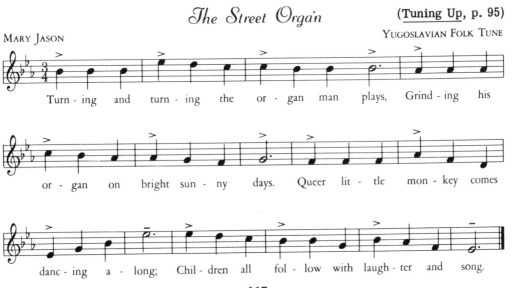

Turn - ing and turn - ing the or - gan man plays, Grind - ing his

or - gan on bright sun - ny days. Queer lit - tle mon - key comes

danc - ing a - long; Chil - dren all fol - low with laugh - ter and song.

Rock-a-by

(Rhythms and Rimes, p. 34)

J. G. HOLLAND

CLARA EDWARDS

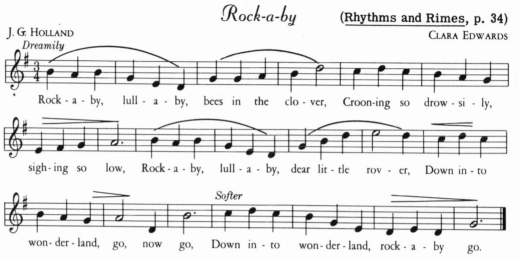

Rock - a - by, lull - a - by, bees in the clo - ver, Croon-ing so drow - si - ly,

sigh - ing so low, Rock - a - by, lull - a - by, dear lit - tle rov - er, Down in - to

won - der - land, go, now go, Down in - to won - der - land, rock - a - by go.

Any other similar songs which begin on the "one" or first beat of the measure may be substituted for these. The children sing with decided accent; they notice that a measure bar occurs before all the strong notes except those at the beginning of a line or staff.

Such questions as the following can be used to give experience in the use of the new terminology:

How many measures are there in the first phrase of the song?
How many notes are there in the first measure of the song?
What words are sung to the notes in the third measure?
What kind of notes are found in the first three measures?
What kind of notes appear in the fourth measure?
How many phrases are there in the entire song?
How many measures are there in the entire song?

(3) DUPLE MEASURE

The same type of experience can be provided with songs in duple measure, such as

Bouncing Ball

(Tuning Up, p. 58)

MARY SMITH

ENGLISH FOLK TUNE

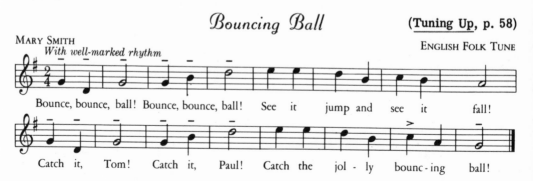

Bounce, bounce, ball! Bounce, bounce, ball! See it jump and see it fall!

Catch it, Tom! Catch it, Paul! Catch the jol - ly bounc - ing ball!

The Violin and the Drum (Rhythms and Rimes, p. 33)

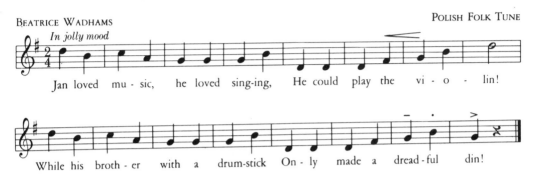

B. UNDERSTANDING THE MEASURE SIGNATURE

For this additional experience the class sings from books a familiar song in 4/4 measure, beginning on the first beat of the measure. The children move their hands silently to indicate the accented and unaccented beats. The following are suggested as typical songs for this step:

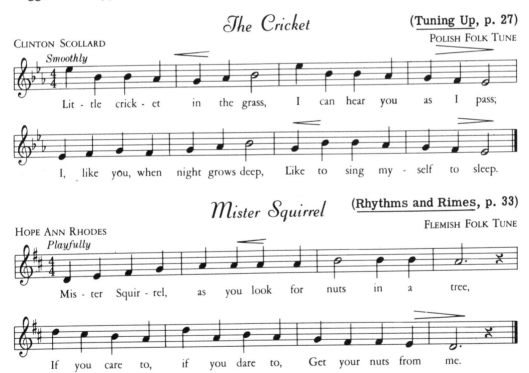

The teacher asks the children to find a measure (or measures) which contain quarter notes only, by means of such questions as the following:

How many quarter notes are there in the first measure? in the fifth measure? As you notice the two numbers at the beginning of the song, what is the upper number of the two?

Without any pause the teacher continues, "Let's look at some other song we know."

The Kind Kangaroo (Tuning Up, p. 16)

MABEL LIVINGSTONE

MANA-ZUCCA

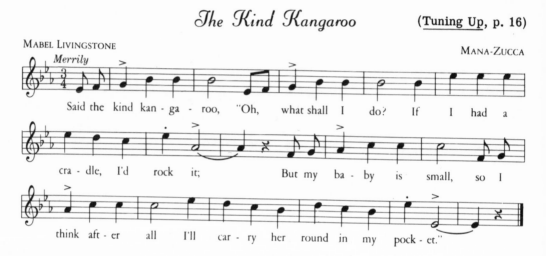

Said the kind kan - ga - roo, "Oh, what shall I do? If I had a

cra - dle, I'd rock it; But my ba - by is small, so I

think aft - er all I'll car - ry her round in my pock - et."

"Rock-a-by" on page 118 may also be used in this connection.

Can you find a measure which has only quarter notes in it?
How many quarter notes does it contain?
What is the upper number of the two which appear at the beginning of this song?

The teacher asks the children to look at other songs they have learned to sing, such as "Bouncing Ball," p. 118, "The Violin and the Drum," p. 119, or any familiar songs in duple measure. They are asked to find

a. Some measures that include only quarter notes
b. The number of quarter notes in each one of these measures
c. The upper number appearing at the beginning of the song.

From a study of these songs or songs similar to them, the class is led to understand that the upper figure indicates the number of quarter notes that make a complete measure. If the three songs in duple, triple, and quadruple measure are available on charts or can be placed beside each other on the blackboard just for this first experience, it will be still easier for the children to see the three contrasting types of measures and the three different measure signatures, and to compare them without going from one to another in a book. It is suggested that, through this approach of allowing the pupils to discover these differences for themselves by means of contrasting song materials, they will readily learn to comprehend the significance of the measure signature. This method will be found far more effective than the customary formal approach in which the teacher simply tells the class that the upper figure indicates the number of beats in each measure, and the rule is memorized.

If the children inquire about the lower number, the teacher can explain that the lower number 4 stands for the quarter note. Therefore, the upper number really tells us how many notes <u>of the kind indicated by the lower number</u> will be needed to <u>fill</u> a measure. Frequently, however, this explanation about the lower number in the signature is best left until a later time. All the songs the children read for some time have 4 as the lower number in the measure signature. When the class becomes definitely curious about the meaning of the lower number, or when they start to read a song having a 2 or an 8 instead of a 4 for a lower number, then they will quickly absorb its significance. Before that time the explanation will probably have little lasting value. If technical points of this kind are introduced <u>when needed</u>, and not before, the whole learning process will be easier.

In this connection, the children will also eventually learn that these two numbers at the beginning of the song are called the <u>measure signature</u>.

Although in these songs used as illustrations the upper number of the measure signature coincides with the number of beats and the lower number agrees with the kind of note that receives one beat, the teacher should realize that this is not always the case.

> For example, in 6/8 measure, there are usually <u>two</u> beats in each measure and not six. Much confusion will result later if the class is taught that the upper number of the measure signature indicates the number of <u>beats</u> in the measure and that the lower number indicates the kind of note that gets one beat. This should not be emphasized. Rather it is important to call attention to the fact that the upper number indicates how many notes of the kind denoted by the lower figure, or the equivalent, will be needed to fill a measure.

C. APPLICATION OF THE MEASURE BAR AND MEASURE SIGNATURE

(1) Before the music period begins, the teacher writes on the board the melody of a <u>familiar</u> song in 2/4, 3/4, or 4/4 measure, <u>without</u> measure bars or measure signature. The following is an example:

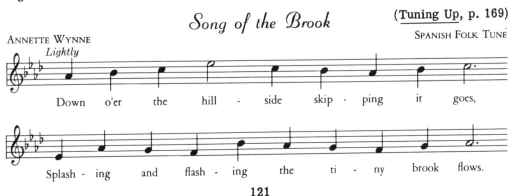

Song of the Brook
(Tuning Up, p. 169)

ANNETTE WYNNE
SPANISH FOLK TUNE

Lightly

Down o'er the hill - side skip - ping it goes,

Splash - ing and flash - ing the ti - ny brook flows.

(2) The children sing the song with words, indicating the accented or strong notes with their hands as they sing. Members of the class show the "strong notes" by putting an accent mark, > , or the letter S over the proper notes in the melody on the board.

(3) When all the "strong notes" have been located and properly marked, some pupil puts in the measure bars, one immediately preceding each strong beat, keeping in mind that when a phrase begins on an accented beat the first bar line is omitted. A double bar, indicating the conclusion of the song, is placed at the end of the second phrase.

(4) The children then notice that three quarter notes fill a measure in this song. The figure 3 is written in the two upper spaces, just before the first note of the first phrase. Some member of the class writes the figure 4 in the two lower spaces, indicating that three quarter notes are required to fill a measure.

The above steps should be taken with at least two other songs, one in 2/4 measure and one in 4/4 measure. The following songs are examples:

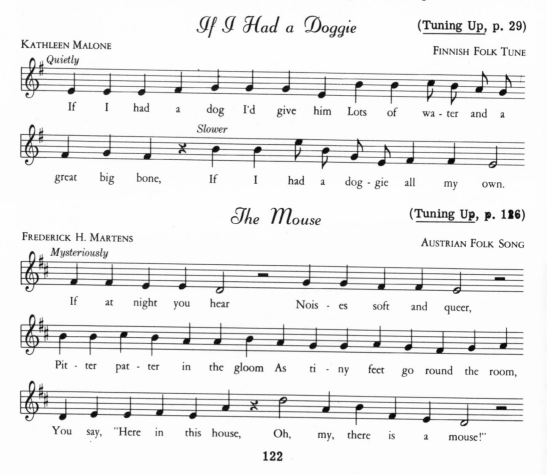

If I Had a Doggie

(Tuning Up, p. 29)

KATHLEEN MALONE

FINNISH FOLK TUNE

Quietly

If I had a dog I'd give him Lots of wa - ter and a

Slower

great big bone, If I had a dog - gie all my own.

The Mouse

(Tuning Up, p. 126)

FREDERICK H. MARTENS

AUSTRIAN FOLK SONG

Mysteriously

If at night you hear Nois - es soft and queer,

Pit - ter pat - ter in the gloom As ti - ny feet go round the room,

You say, "Here in this house, Oh, my, there is a mouse!"

Any similar songs from the books which the class is using may be substituted. The attention of the class should be called to any quarter (one beat) and half (two beat) rests that occur in these songs.

The children should learn also that the measure signature is sometimes used instead of 4/4. The following is an example:

Christmas Windows

(Tuning Up, p. 83)

MARY JASON

GERMAN FOLK TUNE

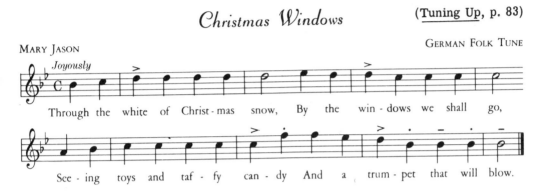

Through the white of Christ-mas snow, By the win-dows we shall go,

See - ing toys and taf - fy can - dy And a trum - pet that will blow.

D. RHYTHM BAND NOTATION SCORES

The rhythm band now progresses to the use of picture scores. These scores, through the use of pictures of the various rhythm band instruments, symbolize measure in music. Each child should have his own part, and play in the measure and on the beats indicated in his part. The children will be able to learn many more selections in this manner, and will greatly enjoy playing from individual parts as real band and orchestra players do.

The teacher's music score and pupils' picture score of the Swedish Folk Dance "Klappdans" follow; also a table explaining the meaning of the symbols.

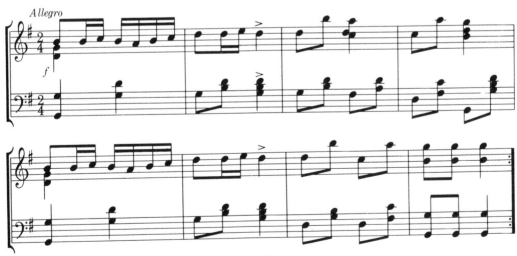

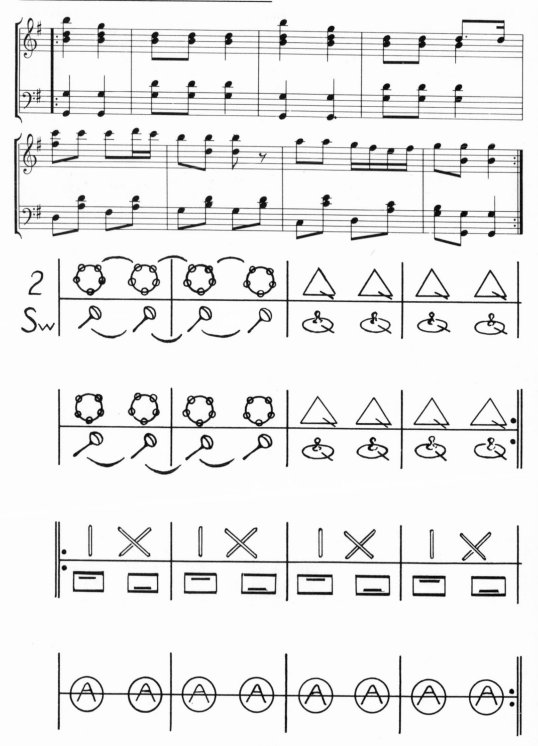

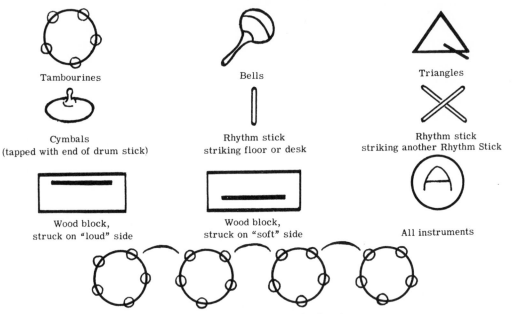

Tambourines

Bells

Triangles

Cymbals
(tapped with end of drum stick)

Rhythm stick
striking floor or desk

Rhythm stick
striking another Rhythm Stick

Wood block,
struck on "loud" side

Wood block,
struck on "soft" side

All instruments

Continuous shake of tambourines for four beats

It is suggested that an enlarged copy of the score be drawn on a single piece of white cardboard large enough to be plainly seen by all pupils.

Chapter XI
Notation of Phrase Rhythms

Before beginning the activities which are outlined in this chapter it is important that the children shall have had ample experience with the activities outlined in the previous chapters, such as recognition of and response to musical phrases, accent, measure signature, and to the rhythmic notation represented by ♩, ♫, ♩♩, ♩, ♩·, ○, ✗ and ━ . The purpose of this chapter is to extend the musical skill and understanding already developed so as to include recognition of and writing of the rhythmic patterns of notes in familiar songs which have been memorized, and also in unfamiliar songs and instrumental music. This recognition and writing is based on the sense of hearing and not of seeing. Even if the pupils in the class have had extensive experience in reading songs, opportunities of the kind outlined here will prove to be an enjoyable "game" approach for developing ear attention. <u>Ear</u> attention to sounds heard, <u>eye</u> attention to notes seen, and a generally improved co-ordination of ear and eye will result in increased skill and musicianship.

1. NOTATION OF PHRASE RHYTHMS IN FAMILIAR SONGS

A. PROCEDURE

All of the work for this phase of development is done without books or music in the hands of the pupils. Only familiar songs are used. It is possible that the children may have learned some of the songs by rote with books open before them or even by reading, but probably they have given slight attention to the values of the notes. This can be real aural work because the rhythmic patterns will seldom be remembered accurately when the books are closed.

The class is being asked now to visualize and write rhythmic patterns of phrases which they have sung and experienced. As a check at the end of the lesson the rhythmic pattern of the phrase which members of the class have just written on the board may be compared with the way the song is printed in the books.

It is suggested that the <u>teacher</u> write the phrase rhythms of the first song on the board in order that the pupils may understand exactly what is expected of them. The pupils will probably wish to write the notes for songs which are used at a later time.

(1) The teacher may select a song that has been memorized and therefore is familiar, such as "Our Flag."

126

Our Flag

(Tuning Up, p. 40)

JANE N. SHELDON

CZECHOSLOVAKIAN FOLK TUNE

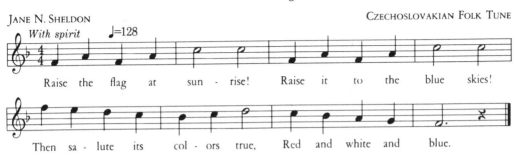

Raise the flag at sun - rise! Raise it to the blue skies!

Then sa - lute its col - ors true, Red and white and blue.

Note. This song is chosen simply because it is the type best suited for this first lesson. The fact that it is taken from a song book designed for a certain grade does not confine this experience to that grade. It is a valuable experience for any grade.

(2) The pupils mark the phrases as they sing the song (see Chapter IV, p. 50) and discover that there are four phrases. The teacher writes the words on the board by phrases, leaving space above each line:

> Raise the flag at sunrise!
> Raise it to the blue skies!
> Then salute its colors true,
> Red and white and blue.

(3) The pupils sing the first phrase of the song, swinging their arms rhythmically to each quarter-note beat as they are accustomed to do (p. 102), and at the same time listen carefully to discover the kind of notes they are singing.

> Teacher: What kind of notes did you sing?
> Pupils: Walking (quarter) notes.
> Teacher: Were all of the notes quarter notes?

If the answer is "Yes," the class sings the phrase again, making rhythmic response. This should cause them to notice that each of the last two notes has two beats and therefore they are half notes.

These notes are then written on the board above the words of the first phrase:

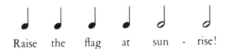

Raise the flag at sun - rise!

The class next sings the second phrase.

> Teacher: What kind of notes did you sing this time?
> Pupils: Just the same as we did with the first phrase.

Again the notes are written above the words of the second phrase:

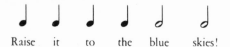

Raise   it   to   the   blue   skies!

In much the same manner the other two phrases are sung from memory and analyzed as to rhythm, and the notes are written <u>above</u> the words:

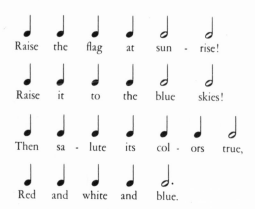

Raise   the   flag   at   sun - rise!

Raise   it   to   the   blue   skies!

Then   sa - lute   its   col - ors   true,

Red   and   white   and   blue.

(4) The pupils now locate and mark the strong notes or "ones" in each phrase with an accent sign (>) and place the measure bars before each accented note, except, of course, when it is the first note in a phrase.

The addition of the measure signature $\frac{4}{4}$ (which really means $^4/\!\!\downarrow$) should be a natural, easy step. It will already be established in the minds of most children both by sensing the accented and unaccented beats in each measure and by looking at the measures written on the board. When this has been done it will usually be wise to erase the accent marks in order to prevent overemphasis of the strong beats when they are marked with these signs.

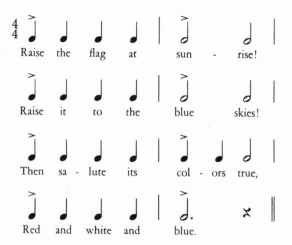

Raise   the   flag   at   sun - rise!

Raise   it   to   the   blue   skies!

Then   sa - lute   its   col - ors   true,

Red   and   white   and   blue.

B. CHOICE OF SONGS

The songs to be used in this connection should be selected carefully. They should be in 2/4, 3/4 or 4/4 measure; the quarter note should always be the unit of beat; and only the rhythmic note patterns thus far introduced should be included.

Notes: ♩ ♩ ♩ ♩ ; ♪♪♪♪ ; ♪. ♪♪. ♪ ; 𝅗𝅥 𝅗𝅥 ; 𝅗𝅥. 𝅗𝅥. ; 𝅝 𝅝 .

Rests: 𝄽 ; ▬ .

Songs used for this purpose should be learned and memorized well in advance of this experience in notating rhythmic patterns in phrases, so that they will be thoroughly familiar to the class. The teacher must be very careful to see that the songs are learned and sung by the class exactly as they are to be written. For example:

♩ 𝄽 should not be sung 𝅗𝅥 or vice versa

𝅗𝅥 𝄽 should not be sung 𝅗𝅥. or vice versa

♪ ♪ should not be sung ♪. ♪ or vice versa

If by any chance a song has been learned incorrectly as far as the rhythmic patterns are concerned, it should not be used for this type of experience.

As additional problems in rhythm, like those presented in the succeeding chapters, are brought within the experience of the boys and girls, songs including new rhythmic combinations, such as ♩. ♪ and compound measure, can be used in a similar way.

2. NOTATION OF PHRASE RHYTHMS IN THE MELODIC LINE OF FAMILIAR INSTRUMENTAL MUSIC

A. PROCEDURE

In addition to writing the rhythmic patterns heard in familiar songs, pupils should also have experience in writing the rhythmic patterns which are found in the melody of familiar instrumental music played on the piano. The class should have heard these selections often enough to be able to remember easily the melodic phrases and the rhythmic patterns they follow.

The procedure in such a lesson will be much like that used when the rhythm of familiar songs is notated, except that there will be no words to serve as a skeleton for the music as it is reconstructed rhythmically.

A familiar instrumental composition such as "To a Wild Rose" (MacDowell) may be played, using only the first theme.

(1) The children listen to the music, indicating the rise and fall of each phrase by the customary movement. When they have discovered the number of phrases, a

129

line (either curved or straight, according to the desire of the class) is drawn on the board for each phrase.

(2) The class next listens to discover the kind of notes that make up the rhythmic scheme of each phrase, taking one phrase at a time, as was done with the notation of songs. The teacher, or some pupil, records the result on the lines on the board. For example, the first phrase of "To a Wild Rose" would appear like this:

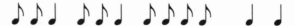

(3) As the music is heard again, the children locate the accents and thus determine where the measure bars belong, and insert them. Finally, the measure is discovered by sensing the strong and weak beats in each measure and by looking at the measures pictured on the board. The final record of the rhythmic pattern of each phrase as it is transcribed will appear like this:

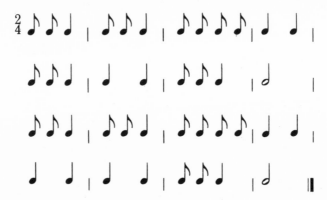

Care must be taken in playing the music to make sure that the left-hand accompaniment is kept subdued. The melody and its rhythmic pattern must stand out clearly and not be complicated by the rhythm of the accompaniment. Where feasible, it is a good plan to have the pupils sing with some neutral syllable the melody whose rhythmic pattern they are to write.

B. CHOICE OF MUSIC

It is important that music selected for these activities be simply and clearly organized as to rhythmic patterns and general structure with a well-defined melodic line, preferably in the right hand. If the selections used have identical rhythmic patterns in both hands, or have the melodic line chiefly in unison, the rhythmic patterns will be easily recognized. The music should be in 2/4, 3/4 or 4/4 measure, and the melody should include only the notes and rests listed under "Choice of Songs" on page 129.

The following selections are suggested as suitable for this experience, and are all found in <u>Play a Tune</u>.

Title	Source	Page
Flora Gave Me Fairest Flowers	English	70
Folk Dance	Danish	25
Musette	Gluck	28
Écossaise	Schubert	30
Nocturne	Chopin	49
Cornelius March	Mendelssohn	37

3. NOTATION OF PHRASE RHYTHMS IN UNFAMILIAR SONGS

Following the writing of the rhythmic patterns in familiar songs, the class may be given an opportunity to discover and write the phrase rhythms of a few unfamiliar, simple songs as they are presented by the teacher. Either of the procedures already outlined may be used: writing the words of the song on the board by phrases and using them as a basis for writing in the different kinds of notes heard; or drawing a straight or curved line for each phrase and using these lines to form a skeleton picture into which the notes heard in each phrase may be fitted. It will be necessary for the teacher to sing the song over and over again while the pupils are discovering the different kinds of notes and writing them. But by the time the lesson is completed the song will be familiar to the class. Songs for such experiences must be carefully chosen, and include only the notes and measure signatures already suggested on page 129. The song books used by the pupils include many songs which are appropriate. In addition, the following standard songs can be used:

> Long, Long Ago
> Are You Sleeping? (Frère Jacques)
> Jolly Old Saint Nicholas
> There's Music in the Air
> The Bluebells of Scotland
> Lightly Row

A little well-directed activity of this sort from time to time will be enthusiastically received by the children, but it is important that such periods be brief and that the music used is not too taxing. If the response of the class is spontaneous the result will be genuine enjoyment, improved musicianship and skill, and also an increase in the accuracy of the singing will be noted.

4. NOTATION OF PHRASE RHYTHMS IN THE MELODIC LINE OF UNFAMILIAR INSTRUMENTAL MUSIC

Very simple phrase rhythms from unfamiliar instrumental selections may also be played, while the pupils listen and then record the rhythmic patterns which they hear. The procedure already suggested on page 129 will be found adaptable for such activities, except that the music, being unfamiliar, may have to be heard more often than was necessary with the familiar tunes. Also, it is possible to profit by listening intensively to certain selected melodies in long compositions, recording the rhythmic patterns whenever the music is heard, without attempting to notate the phrase rhythms of the entire composition. It is possible to use the piano or some other solo instrument or even a phonograph record on which the melody can be clearly distinguished for this experience. Children who are good enough musicians can play their own instruments while the rest of the class listen, sometimes for passive enjoyment and sometimes for active attention to rhythmic patterns and measure signatures. In a similar way, the pupils will frequently enjoy transcribing for their own notebooks the rhythmic patterns of prominent melodies in the music they hear in their listening lessons. These transcriptions of rhythmic patterns are possible where wide range of melody or many changes in key make it impractical to attempt to record the tune melodically.

Each of the following selections includes several phrases suitable for recording phrase rhythms in unfamiliar instrumental music:

Amaryllis	Ghys
Andante (Surprise Symphony)	Haydn
Melody in F	Rubinstein
Chanson Triste (Opus 40, No. 2)	Tchaikovsky
Melody of Love (first theme)	Engleman
The Secret	Gauthier
Minuet in G	Bach
Serenade Badine (middle section)	Gabriel-Marie
Cradle Song	Hauser

As the children increase their rhythmic vocabulary with the experiences of the succeeding chapters, it will be possible for them to use music including many additional rhythmic patterns, thus permitting a wider variety of music for the activities described in this chapter.

Chapter XII
Reading Rhythms in Unfamiliar Music

The prerequisite for the activities presented in this chapter is the same as that given in Chapter XI. Pupils need to have an extensive experience with the recognition, by sight and by ear, and ability to respond to ♩, ♫, ♫., ♩, ♩., ○, ♩, — and — in 2/4, 3/4 or 4/4 measure. Some of the activities described herein can be started after considerable experience of the type suggested in Chapter VIII, p. 88. However, the response will be more spontaneous and enjoyable if preparation is made through the experiences outlined also in Chapter IX, X and XI.

The purpose of the suggestions contained on the following pages and the activities associated with them is to enable the children to make definite application of the rhythmic skills and experiences thus far acquired in the independent reading of new, unfamiliar music.

1. READING RHYTHMS IN UNFAMILIAR SONGS

A. CHOICE OF SONGS

The new songs to be used for these activities should be carefully selected. They should contain only the rhythmic combinations of note and rest values with which the pupils have had experience thus far. These are listed in the first paragraph of this chapter.

B. SUGGESTED PROCEDURES

The children open their books to an unfamiliar song, such as the following:

Wooden Shoe Dance (Rhythms and Rimes, p. 99)

MARCHETTE GAYLORD CHUTE

SWEDISH FOLK TUNE

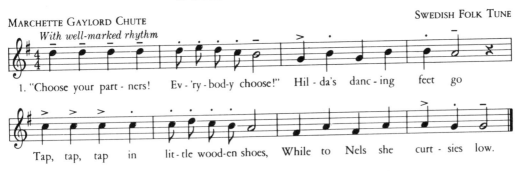

1. "Choose your part - ners! Ev - 'ry - bod-y choose!" Hil - da's danc - ing feet go

Tap, tap, tap in lit - tle wood-en shoes, While to Nels she curt - sies low.

133

LEARNING MUSIC THROUGH RHYTHM

The following questions will direct attention to the rhythmic notation:

How many kinds of notes are there in the song?
What kinds of notes do you see?
Are there any rests?
Can you find two phrases or lines which contain the same combination of notes
　or rhythmic patterns?

After this introductory survey of the music any one of the following four methods of response may be used. It should be borne in mind that whenever children are asked to read the notation of rhythmic patterns, the teacher should establish the tempo before they start. She may count or give her directions rhythmically, chanting the words at the correct speed in this manner:

For duple measure:　　　One, two, / one, <u>read</u> (or <u>sing</u> or <u>play</u>)
　　　　　　　　　　　　　　　　　　or
　　　　　　　　　　　Here we / go, <u>read</u> (or Here we / start, <u>read</u>)
For triple measure:　　One, two, three, / one, two, <u>read</u> (or any other words
　　　　　　　　　　　to give directions and tempo simultaneously.)
For quadruple measure:　One, two, three, <u>read</u> (or words as above)

It is frequently still more satisfactory if the teacher simply taps these preliminary beats, instead of counting or chanting, to set the tempo and then start the group into action by only one word, such as <u>read</u>, <u>sing</u>, <u>play</u>, etc.

If the music begins on some beat other than the first one in the measure, the teacher will speak the word of direction (<u>read</u>, <u>sing</u>, <u>play</u>) on the beat before the one on which the class is to begin.

(1) BODILY RESPONSE TO THE PHRASE RHYTHM

As an introductory question the teacher may ask, "Who can step the rhythm of the first phrase?" Several children are given the opportunity to step this phrase rhythm. They may do this

a. From memory, after a quick glance.
b. With book in hand.
c. From the notation of the phrase rhythm on the board.

The succeeding phrase rhythms of the song are stepped in the same manner.

(2) READING WORDS OF PHRASES IN THE RHYTHM OF THEIR NOTATION

The children are asked to read the words of the song silently from their books until they are thoroughly familiar with them. Strange or unusual words should be pronounced and their meanings explained.

Individual pupils then read the words of the song to the rhythm of their notation, showing the measure, strong and weak beats, with the arm. See Chapter VIII,

p. 91. As each child reads aloud, the class reads silently with him to see that he fits the words of the song correctly to the rhythmic pattern of the notes. As a rule he should be allowed to finish the song before mistakes are corrected. If, however, he reads the rhythm incorrectly in almost every measure, it will be better to call on someone else in order to prevent the incorrect phrase rhythm from being heard too often.

If the class has had experience in reading the melody as well as the rhythmic pattern of the music, the pupils may now read the melody of the song by syllable or number, or whatever method they have learned to use. Otherwise the tune itself may be learned by rote. Many classes are capable of reading rhythm independently long before they can read the melodic line. It will be found that a previously acquired familiarity with the reading of rhythm will make it much easier for children to read the musical score when they begin melody reading.

The teacher is cautioned against too frequent use of the device of chanting the words rhythmically without singing them on pitch. It sometimes retards the development of children who are still in the process of learning to sing a melody accurately, making them feel that the song moves along rhythmically, but in a monotonous chant rather than as a definite melody with tones moving up and down on varying pitches. Overemphasis of rhythmic chanting may make such children so accustomed to producing these monotonous effects with their voices that their attempts to sing melodies will be seriously affected. Vocal rhythm reading should seldom be an isolated activity. Every song which is read rhythmically (whether with words, music syllables, or neutral syllables) should be learned at once, either by reading or rote, or by a combination of the two through the use of diminishing teacher aid.

(3) READING PHRASE RHYTHMS WITH A NEUTRAL SYLLABLE

Pupils who have not yet acquired much skill in language reading may have difficulty with some of the preceding activities. In such cases it is suggested that the class read the phrase with some neutral syllable, perhaps an imitation of the sound of an instrument. For example, they may read the rhythm using the syllable "tah" in imitation of a trumpet, "too" in imitation of a flute, or "pah" in imitation of a trombone. After the children have read the rhythm correctly and have it well in mind, they may attempt the words.

(4) PLAYING PHRASE RHYTHMS

For the sake of variety, children enjoy using the edge of the desk as a piano keyboard while reading or singing phrase rhythms from their books. Drums and other percussion instruments may be used also. Not all of them produce the sustained sound of the half, dotted half, and whole notes satisfactorily; however, if the voice accompanies the playing, either by chanting or singing, the feeling for the duration of longer notes will easily be kept.

2. THE USE OF RHYTHMIC NOTATION AND THE RHYTHM BAND

A. GENERAL PROBLEMS

The class is now ready to make the transition from playing rhythm instruments by rote, by ear, and from picture scores to playing from rhythmic notation. Scores for rhythm bands are available at several publishing firms and are very valuable at this stage of rhythmic study. These scores contain separate parts for the various rhythm instruments. The measures and the note and rest values thus far introduced are used, plus full-measure rests and even rests several measures long.

Most classes are much interested to make the acquaintance of the whole rest ▀▬. Older boys and girls will also wish to know that this rest may be used for any full measure of rest, regardless of the measure signature of the music. They also enjoy learning to count out, two, three or more measures of rest, ⊢²⊣, especially when they understand that most players in real orchestras and bands, particularly those playing percussion instruments, have to count many measures of rest in certain instrumental compositions.

This activity of music reading by using the rhythm band is strongly recommended, especially in the third and fourth grades and later, since it reinforces the reading of both vocal and instrumental music.

When playing from parts scored for the rhythm band, the pupils should be encouraged to exchange instruments freely in order that they may have the experience of playing the varied rhythms which characterize the different groups of instruments.

B. NOTATING ORIGINAL SCORES FOR RHYTHM BAND

The teacher may make her own arrangements for the instruments, choosing suitable selections for the children to read. After some experience in playing from rhythm scores, the children enjoy learning how to notate the original scores they make for themselves. These arrangements made by the children should be kept simple, with few rhythms or parts, and the music used should be rhythmically smooth and easy to follow. If the pupils have had some experience with the making of original orchestrations for rhythm instruments (p. 108) and with notating phrase rhythms, (p. 88) they will easily make the scores for some of their own numbers.

136

When an original score is to be developed, the melody of the music to be used is written on the board, and under this is drawn a line for each group of instruments for which a separate part is to be written. Then one group of instruments, perhaps the jingle group, plays with the music, which may be sung by the teacher or played on the piano. Different members of the class suggest rhythmic patterns which are suited to this group of instruments, and the class chooses the rhythm which seems the best. The notation for this rhythm is written on the board. Then the tinkle group takes its turn, playing different rhythmic patterns to the same music, sometimes alone with the music and sometimes with the first group, until its special pattern is chosen and notated. The third group or any other groups of instruments proceed in the same way until the score is completed. At first the teacher will probably write in the notes, but before long members of the class will be able to do the writing for themselves.

After the score has been completed, a sufficient number of separate parts can be copied to supply the entire class, and the children will enjoy playing their original band arrangements. This type of activity gives opportunity for individuals who are interested in extra music projects; some will make original scores for the class to play, while others will enjoy copying the parts for numbers which are orchestrated. Special orchestrations to produce certain effects or to illustrate the use of instruments that are characteristic of certain countries will be a direct outgrowth of this creative work.

Chapter XIII
Suggestions for Writing the Notation
of an Original Song
Created by the Class

Experiences of the various types outlined in previous chapters, with special emphasis on the activities described in Chapter XI, are a necessary preparation for the work now under consideration. In addition, it is important that the pupils have a broad background of experience in singing and in creating original songs or tunes. With such a foundation of melodic and rhythmic experience the children will be able to do this type of creative work in a way that will make it one of the most purposeful, musically instructive, and enjoyable activities in elementary school music.

These activities may be successfully carried on in many third grades, and will be extremely interesting also in the fourth, fifth, and sixth grades. In order to carry on the work successfully, it is important that the teacher be able to write down accurately the phrase rhythms in the various measures created by the children, and also to notate the melodies they invent after the rhythm has been agreed upon.

A. PROCEDURE

(1) The words of a couplet (two-line poem) are written under a staff on the blackboard. It may be necessary for the teacher to provide the first couplet that is used, but frequently the class or certain individuals will delight in creating original lines to be set to music.

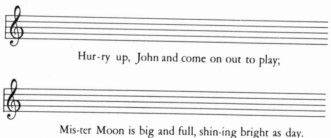

Hur-ry up, John and come on out to play;

Mis-ter Moon is big and full, shin-ing bright as day.

(2) The children read the couplet <u>silently</u> to discover the accented words or syllables. It is important that the reading be done silently, in order to prevent any individual child who is a strong leader from influencing the other children with his chosen rhythmic scheme, as is sure to happen if he reads out loud. There will be

a number of possible plans for accenting the words, and if the class reads the couplet silently several times, individuals will discover these different rhythmic patterns and be able to read them aloud to the group.

(3) Different pupils read the lines aloud to the class to show the accented and unaccented words as they feel they should be. It will be advisable for each pupil, as he reads, to indicate the rhythmic scheme he has chosen by swinging his arms silently in response to the reading, just as he does in response to the music in singing. This will help him to produce a clear demonstration of the rhythmic pattern he has chosen so that others can sense it. As each individual expresses his personal idea, the class reads the words aloud after him. When all suggested plans have been heard and tried, the class chooses the one best liked by the majority.

(4) The pupils now read the words out loud, using the rhythmic scheme they have chosen and indicating the beats by the swinging of the arms. Meanwhile, one child draws a line under each accented word or syllable, like this:

> Hur - ry up John and come on out to play;
> Mis - ter Moon is big and full, shin - ing bright as day.

Or the class may feel that the accented words and syllables should be like this:

> Hur - ry up John and come on out to play;
> Mis - ter Moon is big and full, shin - ing bright as day.

Or possibly they will prefer to accent the word "on" instead of "come" in the first line. The first plan will call for duple measure, the second for quadruple measure.

(5) Another child now places measure bar lines on the staff just before each accented word. If the error is made of placing a bar before the first strong beat in a line of music, attention is called to the fact that if the note following the clef sign is accented, no bar line is placed before it. Since the second phrase begins on an accented word, the last measure of the first phrase is complete and therefore a bar line is placed at the end of the first phrase. A double-bar is placed at the end of the song.

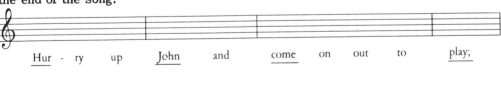

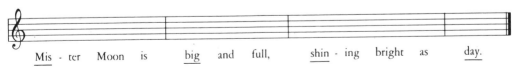

LEARNING MUSIC THROUGH RHYTHM

(6) Using the methods learned in the activities of Chapter IX and X, the class indicates the strong and weak beats by swinging the arms silently as the words are read in the rhythm agreed upon. By counting the number of <u>strong</u> and <u>weak</u> beats between the bar lines, pupils discover the number of beats in each measure. A child then places this number in the upper two spaces of the staff, a little to the left of the first word of the song.

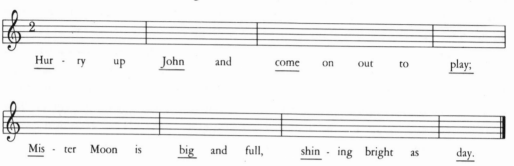

If the class has chosen to accent only four syllables (see paragraph 4, second plan) then there will be only four measures in the song; each measure will have four beats, and so the upper figure will be "4".

(7) The children read the first line of the couplet once more to discover the phrase rhythm. Do the words suggest "walking" notes (quarter notes), "running" notes (eighth notes), or some other kind of notes? One child writes the notes below the words of the first phrase. If preferred, the notes may be written above the staff. The second phrase in turn is read rhythmically, and the notes are written in by another child. If the children swing their arms to indicate the beats as they read, they will recognize that the quarter or "walking" note is the beat note, and therefore the figure "4" should be placed under the "2" to complete the time or measure signature. The rhythmic plan for both phrases now appears as follows:

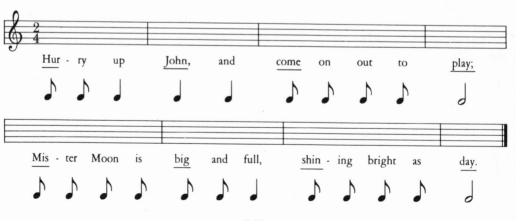

(8) Before this time many classes will have created a melody as well as a rhythm to fit these words. If they have not, however, they should now make up a tune for these words, following the rhythmic pattern recorded on the board. Sometimes this will be done one phrase at a time, and sometimes the entire melody will be produced as a unit by one child. Each pupil who has a tune to suggest sings it to the class, while the teacher records it quickly for her own use. She may write down the notes on the staff, or she may write syllables or numbers, whichever method is most accurate and expeditious. When all the original melodies have been sung by the individuals who created them, and the teacher is confident that she has transcribed them correctly in written form, she may sing each tune to the class, using the words. The class listens and votes to choose the tune best liked. The teacher can easily influence the choice by her comments: "Don't you like this one?" "Isn't this a lovely melody?" or "Do you notice how well this tune seems to fit the words?" In this way, if the teacher so desires, she can lead the group to choose one of the better tunes. Most classes, however, especially as they grow in experience of this kind, will also grow in musical taste and ability to distinguish which tunes are the most attractive and such recognition helps them to choose the best melody.

(9) If the tune created in this way is made up of a melodic vocabulary which the pupils can easily recognize, they may be able to sing it by syllable or number after they have heard it a few times. If they are able to do this they can also, with the assistance of the teacher, then place the note heads on the proper lines and spaces. It is desirable for the teacher to indicate the location of one or do before any attempt is made to notate the melody. In the beginning the teacher will probably have to do much of the writing. But pupils should be encouraged to notate the melody as soon as possible.

One class of children created the following melody for these words. Another class may invent something entirely different, just as they may choose a different rhythmic pattern.

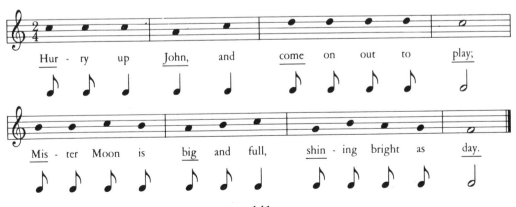

LEARNING MUSIC THROUGH RHYTHM

If the tune created for these words includes unfamiliar skips and tonal groups, or accidentals, so that the class is unable to recognize the notes by ear easily, the teacher should put in the note heads herself. In such cases the children will probably give little assistance except where there are tonal groups that are a part of their musical vocabulary. This is likely to be true particularly with classes of young children or classes where little or no melody-reading has been done as yet. If the children are asked to do only those things which they are ready and able to do easily, all of these steps will be accomplished quickly, and the contribution of the class will be spontaneous. When the work slows down and becomes drudgery, it is usually because it requires skill beyond that which the majority of the members of the class possess. As the experience of the class becomes greater, the skill will also increase. The wise teacher will be content to be ready to do most of the technical transcribing of the melody, encouraging rather than driving the pupils to do more and more as they are able.

(10) Let the children supply the stems to the note heads. In order to do this they will need to know

> (a) On which side (left or right) of the note to place the stem.
> (b) Whether the stem goes up or down.
> (c) How long to make the stem.
> (d) How to make the "flags" or "hooks" on <u>running</u> notes.

They have already learned some of these facts, but they can review and also increase their understanding by examining the notes in the songs in their books. They will see

> (a) That the stems on notes above the third line are on the <u>left</u> side of the note head and extend downward.
> (b) That the stems on notes below the third line are on the <u>right</u> side of the note head and extend upward.
> (c) That the stems on notes written on the third line may extend down or up, depending on the direction of the stems on the neighboring notes.
> (d) That the stem is usually made long enough to pass through three lines or three spaces.
> (e) That the flag or hook is always on the <u>right</u> side of the note stem.
> (f) That the flags extend upward if the stems extend downward, and extend downward if the stems extend upward.
> (g) That the flags pass through approximately two spaces or two lines.

These items of information are interesting to most children. Some will master them and do good work in writing notes accurately. Others will take only a brief interest in the subject. But all will profit by giving attention to it, and will be more intelligent music readers as a result of the experience. The teacher should not be unreasonably exacting in the matter of writing notes, stems and flags, since the object of this activity is not to develop ability to print music. The result should be legible, but not necessarily a work of art.

The teacher may put in the key signature or, if the pupils have the required background in understanding keys, she may lead them to discover for themselves the proper key signature. Such a question as this: "Can anyone tell by singing this melody where 'one,' or do, is located?" Many times this will be discovered through the sequence of notes in the last two measures. In this song, the answer will be, "On the first space." With "one" or do located correctly, many classes will be able to put in the key signature from memory, or by using some rule which has been learned. Others may profit most by finding a song in their books which has the same "one" or do and getting the proper key signature from it.

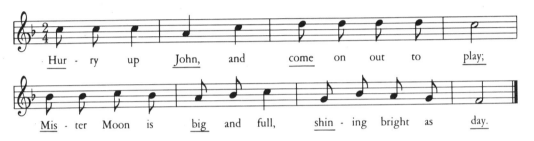

(11) This original composition of the class can now be copied by the teacher and saved for future singing, for display in the classroom, for school exhibits, for the bulletin board, or for other purposes. Some pupils will want to make copies for themselves.

B. CHOICE OF RHYTHMIC PATTERN

A caution concerning rhythmic patterns and how to choose them is timely. Some children will create a tune which uses a rhythmic figure or a measure signature which is foreign to their experience in music reading. For example, consider the following couplet:

> "High up in the tree-tops, snug and warm,
> Mother bird and babies sleep safe from harm."

One child may suggest the following rhythm:

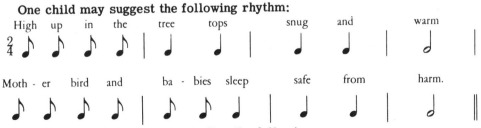

Another child, however, may offer the following:

143

High   up   in   the   tree - tops   snug   and   warm

Moth - er bird   and   ba - bies sleep   safe   from   harm.

Since the rhythmic experiences of the class thus far have included no music except that using the quarter note as the unit of beat and the second rhythmic arrangement above uses the dotted-quarter note, the teacher may find it expedient to encourage the class to choose the first plan suggested. When the children are in the intermediate grades, however, and if they have had a good background of reading rhythmic patterns using the quarter note as a one-beat note, such a situation may offer an ideal opportunity for a clever teacher to introduce 6/8 measure and its beat unit of ♩. as suggested on page 156.

Chapter XIV
The Rhythmic Figure ♩. ♪ in Music,
Using the Quarter Note
as the Beat Note

It is not essential that all the activities presented in the previous chapters be completed before starting the work outlined in this chapter, since some of the earlier experiences may be carried on simultaneously with those suggested here. However, before the activities of this chapter are initiated, it is important that the pupils should have had wide experience with much of the work of the previous chapters and be able easily to recognize, respond rhythmically to, and use in song-reading various combinations of ♩ , ♫ , ♪♪ , ♩ , ♩. , 𝅝 , 𝄽 and ▬ in music in 2/4, 3/4 and 4/4 measure.

In many schools the activities of this chapter will be carried on in the third and fourth grades, but they can begin just as satisfactorily in Grade V or Grade VI. In any case, they should be continued through these grades, or at least until the pattern ♩. ♪ as a musical unit has become an old friend, readily used and interpreted.

A. CHOICE OF MUSIC

Music in which the quarter note is the unit of beat, probably in 2/4, 3/4 and 4/4 or C measure, must be used for the activities presented in this chapter. Music in 3/8, 4/8, 6/8, 9/8, or 12/8 measure must not be used, since the quarter note is not the beat note in these measures. In slow music having these measure signatures the beat note is usually the eighth note, and when the tempo is rapid in 6/8, 9/8, or 12/8 measure the dotted-quarter note serves as the beat or "walking" note.

Music in 2/2, 3/2, 4/2, or ¢ measure can seldom be used for the experiences described in this chapter, since the beat note is usually ♩ , and the figure to be studied, ♩. ♪ , becomes the combination used for skipping, similar to ♩. ♪ when ♩ is the beat note.

B. PROCEDURE

(1) PREPARATORY WORK

Several songs in which the quarter note serves as the unit of beat and which contain the figure ♩. ♪ are learned by rote previous to the first lesson. Such songs as the following from the pupils' books are suggested to serve as <u>introductory</u> or <u>pattern</u> songs:

America
All Through the Night
America the Beautiful
God of Our Fathers

(2) PROCEDURE I: THE FIRST LESSON

The class sings from memory one of the pattern songs, probably "America." No mention has been made of the notes which are to be studied, but the teacher suggests that, as they sing, the children clap with the music, one clap for <u>each note</u> sung.   At the end of the song a brief discussion will reveal the fact that the pupils have recognized both by ear and by muscular feeling that some of the music for certain words was "uneven," "jerky," "skipping," etc. The books are opened to the song, and again the class sings and claps, giving special attention to the music and words which sound uneven. The children discover that the music in these uneven places includes ♩. ♪ in each case.

The pupils will notice as they clap to the song once more that they always have an inclination to give an extra swing or sway between the long note, ♩. , and the short note, ♪.   Since they are already familiar with other dotted notes through previous experience with ♪. ♪ and ♩., they can be expected to recognize that ♩. will be of longer duration than the familiar ♩ or walking note. The impulse to give an extra swing or sway between ♩. and ♪ is simply a natural rhythmic response to the extra length of the dotted-quarter note. It is important to capitalize on this natural impulse and have the class develop a definite feeling for ♩. ♪ by clap, swing, clap-clap.   The <u>sound</u> of the clapping is essential to the development of ability to recognize by <u>ear</u> the uneven rhythmic pattern of ♩. ♪, but the extra <u>silent swing</u> is vital to sustain the muscular feeling for the regular beats in the music. If the children are to make their rhythmic reading accurate they must have this muscular response to guide them.

No study need be made of the mathematical value of the dotted-quarter and eighth-note group. If the children already have a well-developed feeling for accurate movement in response to music, and if they can learn to feel through muscular movement the rhythmic pattern of ♩. ♪, they will read music including such rhythms long before they can intellectually sense the arithmetical use of the dot after the quarter note. It is true that most children can be led, through careful explanation, to understand this musical mathematics. But this intellectual approach does not in any way assure a speedy rhythmic response of the voice when the notes appear in a song which the class is reading. If the ear and muscles are

146

trained to recognize and produce such rhythms when seen by the eye, the intellectual understanding will follow as a natural result for those children who are capable of acquiring it. The series of game drills suggested in paragraph 4 will make it possible to acquire skill with this rhythmic problem in an enjoyable and constantly varied fashion.

It is not necessary to "step" this rhythm. If the teacher or pupils desire to do so it can be done, but such procedure is likely to develop into a complicated dance routine which becomes an end in itself rather than a means of cultivating skill and understanding of the music.

(3) PROCEDURE II: ALTERNATE FIRST LESSON

The class sings one of the familiar songs, with books open, silently marking the beats in the music. They discover as they sing that they are beating twice for the ♩. and that the ♪ is sung after the second beat, and before the beat which follows. In other words, the ♪ is sung between beats. It may help to think of the ♪ in this rhythmic figure as a "slip-in" note. The ♩. , in music which uses the quarter note as the beat note, is therefore to be considered as a two-beat note and not as a beat-and-a-half note. This misconception with regard to this rhythm is generally caused by confusing the idea of beats or pulses in music with the arithmetical value of the notes.

(4) LATER DRILLS

For all of these special drill games it is important that the music used be in 2/4, 3/4, or 4/4 measure in which ♩ is the beat note, and that it contain the rhythmic figure ♩. ♪ as well as notes and rhythmic patterns already familiar. A list of these is given on page 145. The dotted-quarter and eighth notes are always used as a one-unit group and never separately for these activities. Real understanding of this type of rhythmic figure requires that the two notes ♩. and ♪ be learned together. Few classes will use all of these drill activities. The teacher should choose those best suited to meet the needs and interests of her group.

(a) PLAYING THE RHYTHM

Most classes enjoy playing music including ♩. ♪ using drums, (real drums, drums made from oatmeal cartons, etc.). The teacher may put a rhythmic sequence of this kind on the board:

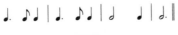

147

LEARNING MUSIC THROUGH RHYTHM

The children play the notes on their drums, striking only once for ♩. but indicating the dot by an extra silent swing away from the drum, followed quickly by the sound for the eighth note. Thus for ♩. ♪♩ the movements would be:

strike   swing   <u>strike</u>   strike

For a ♩ the movements would be strike, swing. For a ♩. the movements would be strike, swing, swing. There should be only <u>one</u> sound for each note. ⅀ represents a regular quarter-note beat, and is played by striking the drum so softly as to produce no sound.

(b) CLAPPING AND CHANTING TO NEW SONGS

Unfamiliar songs in 2/4, 3/4, and 4/4 measure using ♩. ♪ and other familiar rhythmic patterns may be read rhythmically. For example "The Troll of the Hill" (Blending Voices, p. 51) may be read with the class clapping the notes. On the measures including the dotted-quarter and eighth notes the response will be

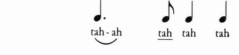

clap, swing   clap clap   clap

It frequently helps pupils to co-ordinate voice and movement if they chant some neutral syllable, such as <u>tah</u> with each note, thus:

tah-ah   tah tah   tah

The Troll of the Hill   (<u>Blending Voices</u>, p. 51)

Translated by
AMY CLARE GIFFIN

NORWEGIAN FOLK SONG

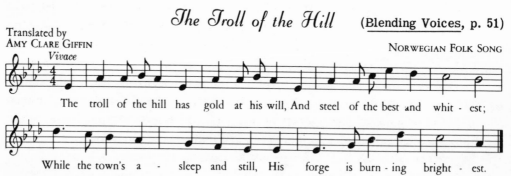

Many other songs which include the rhythmic pattern ♩. ♪ will be found in <u>Songs of Many Lands</u>, beginning on page 74. In <u>Blending Voices</u> suitable songs for developing this rhythmic figure will be found on pages 9, 10, 12, 54, 57, 93, 101, 130, 146, 147, 156, 168, 178, 184, and 188. In <u>Tunes and Harmonies</u> additional unison songs containing this rhythmic pattern are presented on pages 10, 11, 22, 93, and 122.

After chanting the notes, the pupils may enjoy reading the words rhythmically. This will often lead to a spontaneous interest in the song which will result in a desire to read the song melodically. Since the rhythmic structure is already familiar, the reading of the melody should not be difficult for a class with the necessary background of melodic vocabulary. Songs too difficult for reading can be taught by rote.

(c) FLASH CARDS AND A SPELLDOWN

Measures or short phrases can be put on flash cards, but each phrase should be a complete little rhythmic sequence including ♩. ♪ in 2/4, 3/4, or 4/4 measure. The class is divided in the same manner as for a spelldown. The leader shows a flash card and indicates how the rhythm is to be read: "clap it," "chant it," (tah, tah, etc.) or "play it on the drum." Anyone making a mistake takes his seat, until a winner is left undefeated.

(d) THE WRITING OF PHRASE RHYTHMS FROM FAMILIAR SONGS CONTAINING ♩. ♪.

The rhythms of phrases from familiar songs such as "America," "All Through the Night," and "America the Beautiful," in which the figure ♩. ♪ occurs, may be sung from memory and the rhythmic pattern written on the board by the pupils or on plain paper at the desks. Staff-lined paper is not necessary. For example, the first part of "America" will be written as follows:

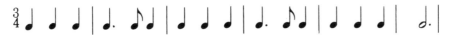

(e) RHYTHMS IN ROUNDS, CANONS, AND PART SONGS

A rhythmic sequence of four to eight measures can be written on the board, or a song from the books may be used. The notes are read rhythmically, either like a round or a canon, by rows or tables. One row starts, playing, chanting, or clapping. One or two measures later, or at a time agreed upon by the group, another row begins, then another and another, until all are participating. It may be necessary to read the entire selection more than once in order to have everyone participating at the same time. This will help develop concentration and a steady rhythm.

The same type of activity can be carried on with two simultaneous parts. Both parts can clap, or chant, or sing, or play, or one part can chant or sing while the other plays an accompaniment. Sometimes several kinds of rhythm instruments can be used in some such form as this:

LEARNING MUSIC THROUGH RHYTHM

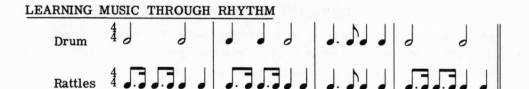

(f) RHYTHM-INSTRUMENT ORCHESTRATIONS

The class will go directly from such a beginning into creative work, with instruments accompanying familiar songs or using original rhythm-instrument scores which include the new pattern ♩. ♪ . For example, one class worked out an original rhythm-instrument accompaniment for "Camp Fire," on page 28 in Blending Voices, as follows:

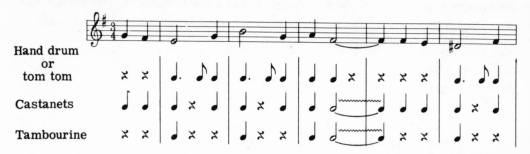

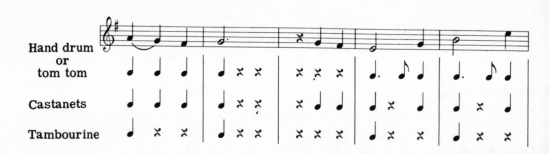

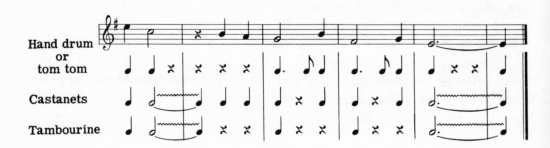

1. By the bonfire's ruddy glories,
   Where the dry logs crack and blaze,
   You shall learn our songs and stories
   And the secret gypsy ways.

2. You may share our ancient learning,
   You may hear our people tell
   How to read the bright stars' turning,
   How to weave a gypsy spell.

3. And if trouble overtake you
   And of city ways you tire,
   You will find all care forsake you
   Here, beside our gypsy fire.

Suggestions for developing such an orchestration are given on page 136.

(g) GAMES

Folk games with music using the rhythmic pattern being studied are invaluable as a means of developing the sure and accurate muscular response so important in this type of experience. One of the most popular games using ♩. ♪ is "The Elephant."

The Elephant

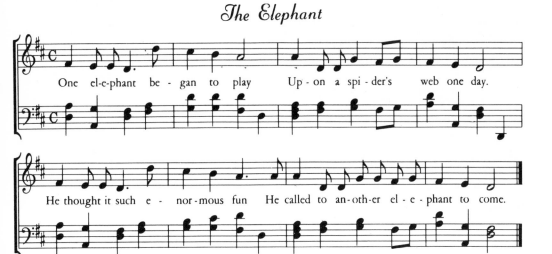

Directions

Formation: One dancer in the middle of the room; the others standing or sitting around the sides.

Figure 1: While all sing, clap, or play rhythm instruments, the dancer in the center, moving in any direction, takes three walking steps forward, starting on the right foot (measure 1, first three beats).

On the fourth beat of measure 1 he stands, and in place points the left foot over the right until the toe touches the floor. Still in place, he steps on

151

the left foot on "-gan" and points the right over it on "to," steps the right foot on the first beat of "play," and points left on the second beat of "play" (measure 2). Starting with the left foot, he takes three walking steps forward and repeats the points as above, but starting with the right toe (measures 3-4).

Repeat Figure 1 (measures 5-8).

Figure 2: Beckoning to a player from around the room, the center dancer performs the above figure as before, but is followed by the person he has invited to join him. This new player places both hands on the hips of his leader and follows his steps closely. Everyone in the room, sings, claps, or plays "Two elephants," etc.

Figure 3: The second player now chooses an addition to the line, and a third person places his hands on the hips of the second dancer and follows closely behind the two others, while all sing "Three elephants," etc. Repeat until the whole group is dancing in line.

If desired, several leaders can start at once in the beginning, thus bringing the entire class into the game very quickly.

This game demands considerable co-ordination; it must be performed with exact rhythm, the same feet in each line pointing in unison. Players will avoid getting their feet tangled if they remember always to take three walking steps before starting the points. A group performing this series of steps together provides a very clever, humorous stunt for a program. This is very usable with older boys and girls, as well as with little folks.

Accompanying Rhythms: Some of the pupils who are clapping or playing rhythm instruments should follow the note line of the song, emphasizing the uneven note patterns. Others should follow the steady rhythm of the steps of the dancers. This will give excellent drill in sensing the use of the dotted quarter followed by the eighth note, since the two rhythms playing simultaneously will be:

| Voices and instruments following melody | ♩ ♪♪♩. ♪ \| ♩ ♩ 𝅗𝅥 etc. |
| Dancer's steps and instruments following the steps | ♩ ♩ ♩ ♩ \| ♩ ♩ ♩ ♩ etc. |

(h) USE OF ♩. ♪ IN THE NOTATION OF ORIGINAL MELODIES.

The class can begin to use the figure ♩. ♪ in the original melodies being composed. It is probable, in a class where much creative work has been done, that this rhythmic pattern has appeared before in original songs which were notated by the teacher. This is the first time, however, that the children have had had ♩. ♪ as a bit of rhythmic vocabulary which they can use consciously and write for themselves. It will be found that the many uses made of this figure in connection with activities presented in this chapter will make it a definite part of the familiar rhythmic vocabulary of the class. They will use it instinctively where it fits the lines being set to music, and will enjoy the increased variety of rhythmic effects it makes available to them. They will soon learn to recognize by ear the swing of lines of poetry that will suggest the use of ♩. ♪ The following lines are parts of poems written by children and illustrate poetic rhythms of the type which may easily be set to music using this figure:

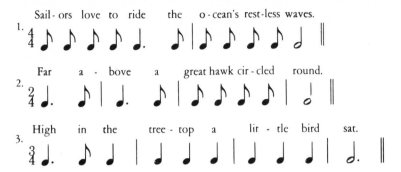

The procedure for developing this creative work is suggested in Chapter XIII.

(i) AURAL RECOGNITION OF ♩. ♪ IN MUSIC HEARD

1. PIANO MUSIC

Further experience in recognizing this rhythmic figure can be gained through the use of piano music which the children hear but do not see. The excerpt from The Merry Wives of Windsor is suitable for such activity. The following rhythmic combinations are placed on the board before the class period begins:

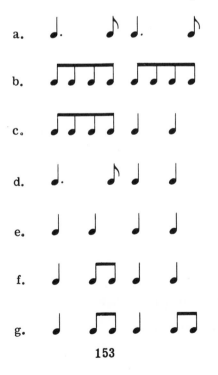

LEARNING MUSIC THROUGH RHYTHM

As the teacher plays the excerpt from The Merry Wives of Windsor, the pupils try to find the different rhythmic patterns which they hear among those on the board.

OTTO NICOLAI

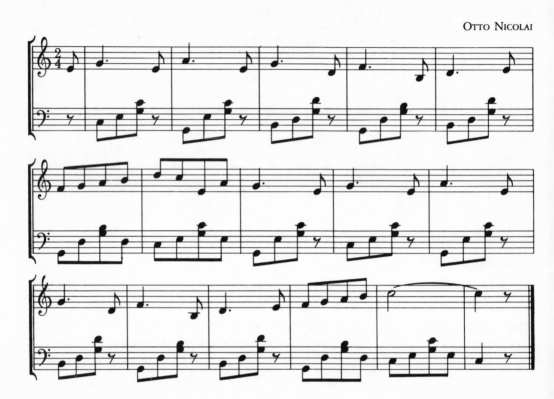

Other similar selections which contain one or more of the rhythms listed should be played. It is important that the music be in 2/4, 3/4, or 4/4 measure with the quarter note as the unit of beat. Sometimes the class will try to decide how many times the figure ♩. ♪ is heard.

(2) SONGS

The teacher plays the song while the pupils look at a list of rhythmic patterns similar to those already given, but including groups from the music being heard. Or part of the class sings while the others watch the notes and count the number of times any of the rhythmic patterns occurs. In addition to the songs listed on page 146, the following are suitable:

> The Harp that Once through Tara's Halls
> Hark the Herald Angels Sing
> Deck the Hall
> Auld Lang Syne

(3) MUSIC IMPROVISED OR ADAPTED

The teacher who can improvise at the piano will find it exceedingly helpful also to play improvisations or to adapt familiar music, as has been suggested in previous chapters, playing one section consisting entirely of two-beat (♩) notes; another section composed of the figure ♩. ♪ ; another of "running" notes, and still another of quarter notes. The pupils are asked to identify, and possibly to write, the kind of notes they hear in the melody or upper part. This aural recognition of rhythmic patterns is a most important phase of ear and eye training.

Chapter XV
The Dotted Quarter Note
Used as the Beat Note in $\frac{6}{8}$, $\frac{9}{8}$, or $\frac{12}{8}$ Measure

Thus far the quarter note has been used as the beat note in the study of rhythmic notation. This is sound music pedagogy because the quarter-note beat is fundamental. Most of the world's music is written with the quarter note as the unit of beat. A great deal of the music sung, played and heard, however, has the dotted-quarter note ($\ ♩.$) as the beat unit, and it is important for the pupils to learn to recognize this type of rhythmic pattern. The purpose of the activities presented in this chapter is to acquaint the class with the manner in which rhythms are written and executed when the dotted quarter note is employed as the unit-of-beat measurement and when the natural division of the beat is in threes ($♪♪♪$) in contrast to the division into twos ($♪♪$), which has become so familiar.

It is important that the class shall have had extensive experience with the activities set forth in previous chapters, especially those in Chapter XIV, before beginning the work outlined on the succeeding pages. In many schools the different experiences which we are about to consider will be conducted for the first time in the fifth grade, but they can begin just as easily in Grade VI or even later if the pupils on these grade levels are not already thoroughly familiar with them.

A. CHOICE OF MUSIC

Only music in 6/8, 9/8, and 12/8 measures should be used for these activities and the tempo should be rapid. There is not as great a quantity of music written in 9/8 and 12/8 measures as there is in 6/8 measure, and therefore more of the latter is included here. Although the tempo of some music in 6/8 measure is slow enough to require and justify six beats to each measure, most of the music with this measure signature should be performed rapidly enough to give the performer and listener the feeling of duple measure, one strong and one weak beat in each measure.

B. PROCEDURE IN THE INTRODUCTION OF 6/8 MEASURE

(1) Several songs in 6/8 measure are taught by rote and thoroughly memorized well in advance of the time when they are to be used as pattern songs for

156

these activities. For classes which use the books of <u>The World of Music</u> the following songs are listed as appropriate for use in this connection:

Blending Voices		Tunes and Harmonies	
Pepita	p. 108	Hiking	p. 46
Jolly Winter	p. 109	Lord Lovel	p. 45
Tomorrow	p. 116	Captain Kidd	p. 98
Trip It Lightly	p. 127	The Valley of Glencoe	p. 59

(2) On the day the rhythmic patterns in 6/8 measure are to be presented, the class sings one of the preparatory or pattern songs, perhaps "Tomorrow," from memory and with books <u>closed</u>. As they sing they swing their arms with the music to discover the number of beats in each measure. They realize that they are beating as follows: <u>strong</u>, weak, <u>strong</u>, weak, etc., or <u>two</u> beats to each measure. It will help the children to recognize this rhythmic pattern by ear if no mention has been made previously of the measure signature or of the subject of the day's lesson. It is important that they sense for themselves that <u>two beats to a measure</u> are clearly defined. The song may profitably be repeated several times to make this muscular response definitely felt.

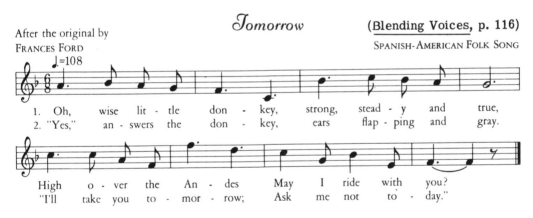

After the original by
FRANCES FORD

Tomorrow

(Blending Voices, p. 116)

SPANISH-AMERICAN FOLK SONG

♩.=108

1. Oh, wise lit - tle don - key, strong, stead - y and true,
2. "Yes," an - swers the don - key, ears flap - ping and gray.

High o - ver the An - des May I ride with you?
"I'll take you to - mor - row; Ask me not to - day."

(3) The books are opened and the children continue to sing and beat time, watching the notes all the while. The teacher says, "We are giving two beats to each measure. Can someone find a measure which includes only two notes?" Two such measures, the second and sixth, with the words "donkey" and "Andes," are discovered, and the pupils notice that each of the notes for each syllable of these two words is receiving one beat as their arms swing rhythmically. Therefore it is apparent that the dotted quarter note receives one beat, or ♩. = 1 beat.

(4) Attention is called to the measure signature, 6/8. In previous experiences the class may have received the impression that the upper figure always indicates

the number of beats in a measure.[1] The pupils will be interested to try beating six beats to a measure as they sing this song. They find that this destroys all the smooth swing of the music. The teacher may explain by saying, "We have discovered that we are really giving two beats to a measure, with a dotted quarter note (♩.) receiving one beat. In the music where a quarter note gets one beat we usually put the figure 4 as the lowest number in the time signature, to indicate this fact. Can anyone think of a number which can be used to represent a dotted quarter note (♩.) in the same way that the 4 represents the quarter (♩) note?" The children discover that the measure signature for this song would be more accurate if it were ²/♩. instead of 6/8. Since there is no number to represent the dotted quarter note, 6/8 is used as a measure signature to indicate how a measure may be filled; that is, music of this kind must have six eighth (♪) notes or the equivalent in each measure.

(5) The teacher continues, "We know that ♩. = 1 beat. As we sing the song again, can you discover any other note or notes used to make up one beat?" The class finds that

$$ \text{♪♪♪ or ♪♪♪} = 1 \text{ beat} $$

$$ \text{♩ ♪} = 1 \text{ beat} $$

"How many beats did you give the dotted half note (♩.) in measure four?" Two. The class sees that the dotted half note fills the entire measure, while in measure eight the pattern ♩.♩ fills <u>almost</u> the entire measure. Such an explanation is sufficiently mathematical for the needs of the average class.

(6) It may help the group in thinking of 6/8 measure as duple or two-beat measure to consider the ♩. as the walking note, ♪♪♪ as the running notes, and ♩ ♪ as the skipping notes, while ♩. is the two-beat note.

Eighth notes were the running notes also in the previous experiences of the class with 2/4, 3/4, and 4/4 measure. It is important that the pupils compare the use of the eighth note in 2/4, 3/4, and 4/4 measures, where there are two running notes to a

[1] "The common teaching that in a meter signature the upper figure denotes the number of beats in a measure, and the lower, the kind of note which has one beat, is only half true. It applies in simple, but not in compound meters. To consider 6/8 as signifying <u>six</u> beats in the measure, with eighth note unit, is to misunderstand the real feeling of duple compound meter. To be sure, in a <u>slow</u> 6/8 measure we may <u>decompose</u> the beat, and feel the <u>background</u> of eighth notes, but this does not make it sextuple meter. It is a duple measure.

"The method of indicating compound meter by signatures seems, perhaps, needlessly complicated. A better signature for 6/8 meter might be 2/4., which shows that there are two <u>dotted quarter notes to a measure</u>. Similarly, 9/8 meter is really 3/4., and 12/8 is 4/4.." From <u>Fundamentals of Musicianship</u>, Vol. I, by Melville Smith and Max T. Krone. Copyright, 1934, by M. Witmark and Sons. Reprinted by special permission.

beat (♫) , with the use of the eighth note in 6/8 measure, where there are three running notes (♫♪) to one beat. Understanding of this fact is essential to the development of skill and ability to read music in 6/8, 9/8, and 12/8 measures.

(7) When the class reviews another familiar song such as "Pepita" (Blending Voices, p. 108), the measures including six eighth notes are discovered. Rather than count "1 - 2, 1 - 2," some children are better satisfied to count "1 - 4, 1 - 4," omitting the intervening beats in a six-beat measure. This may be confusing to many in the class, however, and will not lead as easily to the reading of music in 9/8 and 12/8 measures as will the definite recognition of the dotted-quarter note (♩.) as the beat unit and the steady count of "1 - 2" to each measure.

As other songs are sung, other combinations of notes and rests will occur and be recognized as a part of the rhythmic vocabulary of this kind of measure, namely 𝄾 𝄿 (♩ ♪), which equals ♩., which equals one beat.

C. DRILL ACTIVITIES IN 6/8 MEASURE

(1) Measures of typical rhythmic patterns with 6/8 as the measure signature can be put on the board for recognition by the class. Here are some examples:

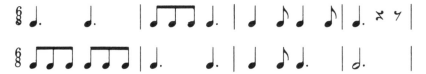

These measures may be read in several different ways.

(a) CLAPPING

The pupils can clap the notes, giving a slight accent to each beat, thus:

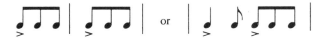

This activity will often bring to light those places where individuals need help. It will also give concrete assistance to those children who lack confidence in themselves, but who can relax and participate when they hear the steady beat of the rhythm when it is produced by the entire group. They also learn through the clapping the necessity for a quick, light, free response to a series of eighth notes such as ♫♩ ♫♩. Children who respond accurately will usually have a tendency to sway slightly to indicate the two beats to each measure and at the same time be clapping lightly with the fingertips for the fast notes.

(b) RHYTHM INSTRUMENTS

Rhythm instruments can be used in the same way. Instruments such as drums, wood blocks, temple blocks, and claves produce a clearer aural representation of this type of rhythm for the first experiences than the rattling or jingling instruments. Before long, however, all types can be used effectively. It is possible to have different groups of instruments representing the varied rhythmic patterns in 6/8 measure and playing simultaneously. This can serve as an illustration:

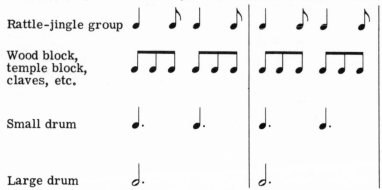

This activity can also be carried on in the form of a round, one instrument starting the rhythmic pattern, another coming in possibly two measures later, then another, and so on. Then on a prearranged signal, the first group stops, the second group stops two measures later, and so on, until only one group is playing at the end.

(c) CHANTING

The children, as they clap, can also chant to these notes, using a neutral syllable, thus:

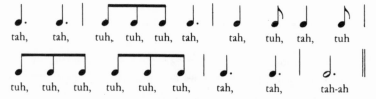

This vocal response to the rhythm is important, because it insures not only an understanding of the notation of the 6/8 measure, but also the ability to reproduce it vocally. Much of the difficulty which pupils experience in reading songs with this type of rhythm is a result of inability to reproduce out loud what is seen and understood, because of lack of skill in co-ordinating the muscles of the voice.

(d) FLASH CARDS

Through the use of flash cards, each with a group of measures which is a rhythmic sequence in 6/8 measure, other drill games can be conducted, including a rhythmic spelldown such as was suggested on page 149.

(2) These same types of activity can be carried on through the reading of new songs in the children's music books. Songs used should include only those rhythmic patterns in 6/8 measure which are familiar or which will be readily understood through previous experience. Some songs in this rhythm are easy to sing when taught by rote, but are much too complicated in their rhythmic patterns for independent reading by any but pupils with a greater musical background and experience than is customarily found in the average child at this age level.

In addition to the various activities suggested in paragraph C, the songs can also be read rhythmically with words. The songs that are in two or three parts will provide interesting ensemble experience through chanting or playing with rhythm instruments. All of these activities provide excellent background for the learning of the melody of the song, either by independent sight singing by the class or by a part-rote-and-part-note process, as is the case with the more difficult songs.

D. 9/8 AND 12/8 MEASURE

In the sixth grade pupils encounter songs in 9/8 and 12/8 measure that move rapidly. These rhythms can be introduced in the same way as was suggested for 6/8 measure. Songs similar to the following from Tunes and Harmonies are suggested for observation and study:

In Days of Old	(fast 9/8)	p. 68
For Our School	(fast 12/8)	p. 100

It is apparent, both on hearing and on looking at songs in 9/8 and 12/8 where the tempo is rapid, that the rhythmic patterns are the same as those in 6/8 measure, with ♩. as the beat unit or walking note. While 6/8 measure is really a duple or two-beat measure, 9/8 is a triple (three-beat) and 12/8 a quadruple (four-beat) measure.

Drill activities similar to those suggested for rhythmic patterns in 6/8 in paragraph C can be used to give further experience with the measure signatures 9/8 and 12/8.

E. LATER EXPERIENCES USING 6/8, 9/8, AND 12/8

(1) THE WRITING OF RHYTHMS FROM FAMILIAR SONGS

The rhythmic patterns of phrases from familiar songs can be written by part of the group while the others sing the songs from memory. The songs appropriate for such use should be in rapid tempo in 6/8, 9/8, and 12/8 measure, in which the dotted quarter note is the unit of beat. The writing can be done at the blackboard or on plain paper. Staff-lined paper is not necessary. If the class is to have the ability to do this easily, it is important that the songs be well memorized before any attempt to recognize or write is made. It will usually help the pupils as they try to hear all the notes clearly if they clap lightly with each word or syllable as they sing. Then they should write the rhythm pattern they have heard and choose the correct measure signature. The first part of "Seesaw, Margery Daw" would be written as follows:

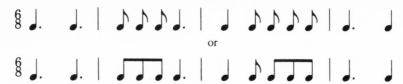

or

Much familiar music has one or another of these measure signatures. Here are some examples:

> Row, Row, Row Your Boat
> Three Blind Mice
> Merrily, Merrily Greet the Morn
> Beautiful Dreamer
> Little Tom Tinker
> Humpty Dumpty
> Rock-a-by Baby
> When Johnny Comes Marching Home
> The Animal Fair
> Oats, Peas, Beans
> The Needle's Eye
> Wild Horseman (Schumann)
> Pop! Goes the Weasel

(2) THE NOTATION OF ORIGINAL MELODIES USING $\downarrow$. AS THE UNIT OF BEAT

The class can now begin consciously to use 6/8, 9/8, and 12/8 measure with the dotted quarter note as the unit of beat in original melodies. If the pupils have done much creative work, doubtless these rhythmic patterns have already appeared in their original songs, but up to this time the teacher has had the responsibility of notating these melodies. After considerable experience of the kind described on previous pages, however, the children will begin to use these new familiar rhythmic patterns spontaneously in their creation of new melodies. Certain poetic rhythms use word and syllable groupings which may be scanned with three short sounds to each rhythmic swing such as ♪♪♪ rather than the two, ♪♪ , to which they have been accustomed up to this point. Music in 6/8, 9/8, or 12/8 measure will be found to fit this type of poetic rhythm most acceptably. Here are a few examples:

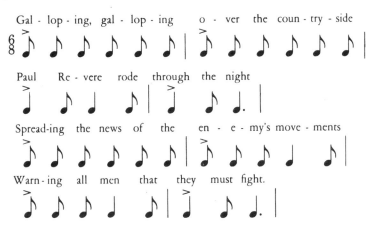

Or the second line might be notated thus:

Some procedures for developing this ability to create or originate tunes are suggested in Chapter XIII. The same ideas can be used here, except that now the dotted quarter note instead of the quarter note functions as the beat unit.

(3) GAMES

Folk games in which the measure signature is 6/8, 9/8, or 12/8 are invaluable as a means of developing sure and accurate muscular response to this kind of rhythm. Such games also increase the feeling for the division of the beat into three parts (♪♪♪) instead of the two parts (♪♪) which have been used so extensively. A popular game which uses this rhythm and is suitable for the pupils is

Push the Business On

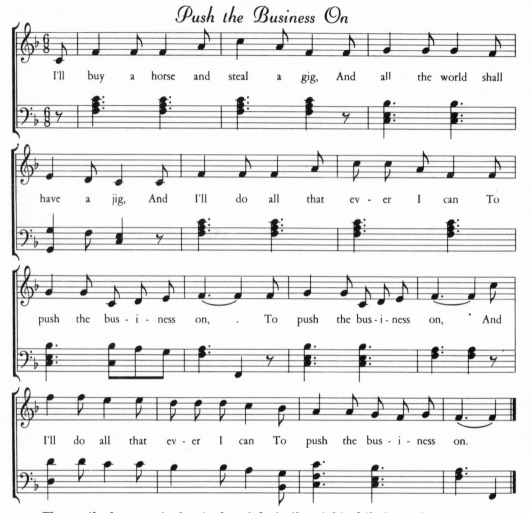

I'll buy a horse and steal a gig, And all the world shall have a jig, And I'll do all that ev-er I can To push the bus-i-ness on, . To push the bus-i-ness on, And I'll do all that ev-er I can To push the bus-i-ness on.

The pupils form a single circle, girls to the right of their partners.

(a) All join hands and move to the right as they sing the first six measures, taking two steps to each measure.

(b) Drop hands. Each dancer turns around in place, clapping his hand four times as he turns. (Measures 7-8)

(c) Partners now face each other, each person clapping his own hands once and his partner's hands three times. (Measures 9-10)

(d) Partners grasp each other's hands and make a complete turn together. (Measures 11-12)

(e) Drop hands. Boys step back; girls take two sliding steps to the left; boys step forward to start the game again with a new partner.

If not all of the children can play this game at the same time, those who listen can orchestrate the music for their instruments, some playing only "1-2, 1-2", and so on, while others play the rhythmic patterns of the notes as they are heard in the music. Then they can sing and play a rhythm-instrument accompaniment for the game.

This is a popular rhythm for games, and many additional familiar games are suggested on page 17.

(4) AURAL RECOGNITION OF RHYTHMIC PATTERNS IN MUSIC HAVING $\downarrow$. AS THE UNIT OF BEAT

Further experience in recognizing the rhythmic figures in piano music can be acquired through the use of instrumental compositions heard by the children but not seen by them. The following rhythmic patterns are put on the board before the lesson begins:

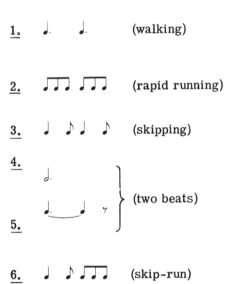

1.   (walking)

2.   (rapid running)

3.   (skipping)

4.   } (two beats)

5.

6.   (skip-run)

As the music for the first selection is played (perhaps "Oats, Peas, Beans," the class identifies the rhythm which is heard by watching the notes on the board. When the music is familiar the pupils will identify a rhythmic pattern more quickly if they clap lightly while listening, since the movement and sound of the clapping accentuate the differences between the groups of notes.

Questions will also help to develop this power of recognition. For instance, "What do you hear in 'Oats, Peas, Beans'?" The answer will be, "Number 3."

"What do you hear in the last measure of this same song?" Answer, "Number 4 or 5."

($\downarrow$.) "Raise your hand if you find the place where there are four walking notes in 'When Johnny Comes Marching Home.' "

"What group of notes do you hear frequently in 'Wild Horseman'?" Answer, "Number 2."

"In how many places do you hear any notes other than ♩♩♪ ♩♩♪ in 'Wild Horseman'?" Answer, "Two."

"Can you find a measure containing 'Number 1' in 'Pop! Goes the Weasel'? How many times is it heard?" Answer, "Two."

The teacher who can improvise at the piano will find it desirable also to play improvisations in 6/8, 9/8, and 12/8 measures in rapid tempo. In these improvisations one section may be composed wholly of skipping notes (♩ ♪) , and other sections of ♩., ♩♩♩ , and ♩. in turn. The pupils can identify or write the notes they hear in the melody (played by the right hand), or upper part. An example of an improvisation follows.

Improvisation

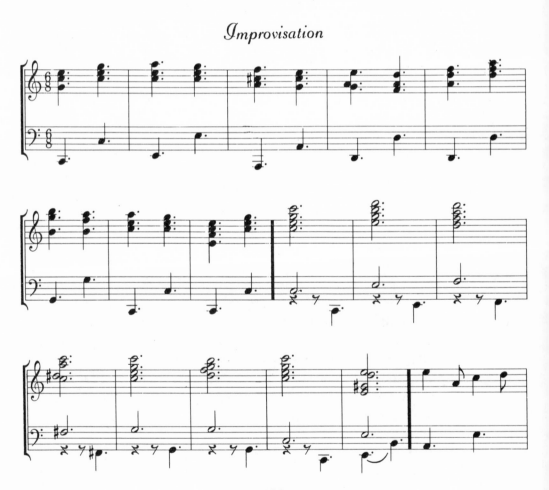

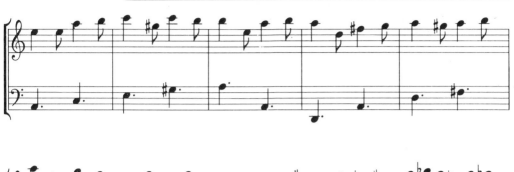

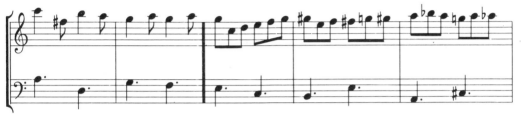

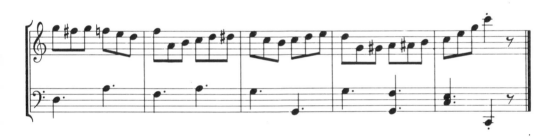

Chapter XVI
Different Kinds of Beat Notes

The material contained on the pages of this book has covered procedures for introducing only the two notes used most commonly as the unit of beat, namely the quarter note (♩) in measure signatures of 2/4, 3/4, and 4/4, and the dotted quarter note (♩.) in 6/8, 9/8, and 12/8 measure. These beat notes are fundamental and the reading of music having the measure signatures listed above should be emphasized in the elementary grades.

In many of the music books which are used in the intermediate grades songs are found where the unit of beat is neither the quarter note nor the dotted quarter note. Also a great many selections for piano, orchestra, and band use some of the common, less familiar beat notes. It is desirable and even essential, therefore, that the pupils become acquainted with other measure signatures and that they be given some experience in reading rhythmic patterns contained in these measures.

A careful study of the following parallel measures and notations of rhythms will clarify this practice for the teacher and should enable her to introduce these additional beat notes so that the pupils will develop some ability and power to read these parallel rhythmic notations effectively.

Songs in simple measure using any one of three different beat notes (♩ , ♩ , or ♪) may be written as follows:

Theme

MOZART

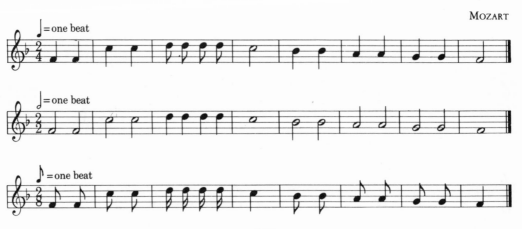

Santa Lucia

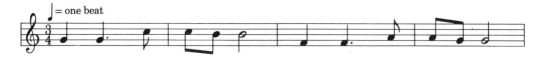

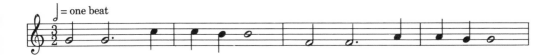

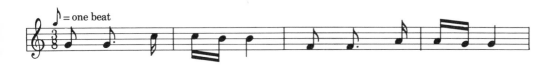

Old Folks at Home

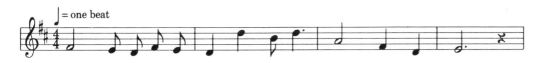

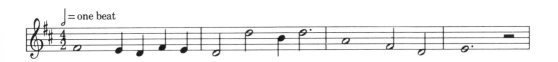

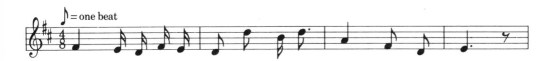

Similarly songs in compound measure may be written using any one of three different beat notes: ♩., ♩. and ♪.

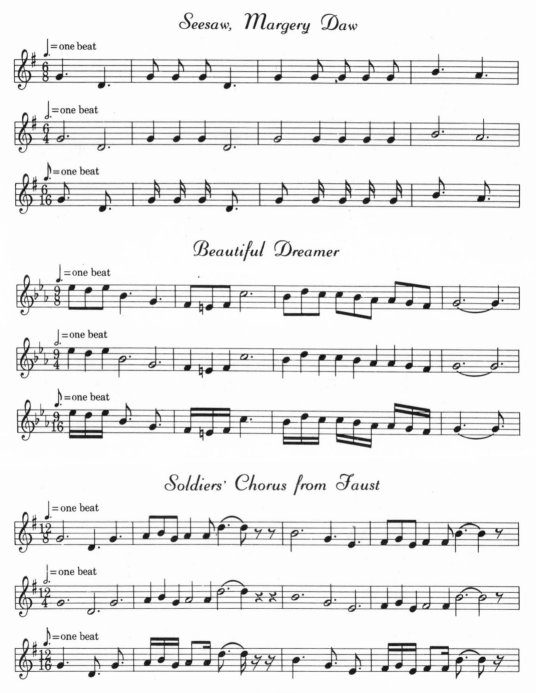

Seesaw, Margery Daw

Beautiful Dreamer

Soldiers' Chorus from Faust

As a means of further assistance in the understanding of parallel notations of rhythms the following "Vocalise" is included here as it would appear if all six beat notes were used. These notations show the use of triplets in simple measures, and the use of duplets and quadruplets in compound measure.

Vocalise (Written in six parallel rhythms)

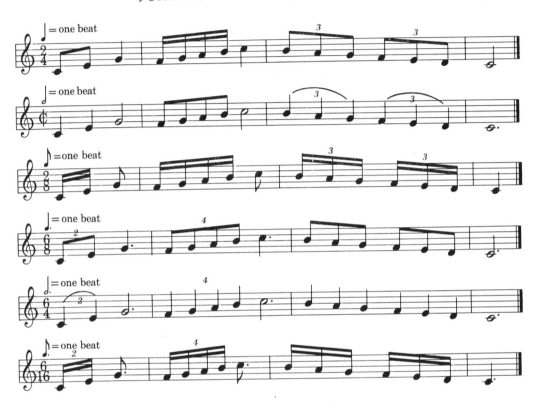

After the teacher has demonstrated how a song or a phrase of a song may be written in several different ways, according to the measure signature and the unit of beat, it is suggested that the pupils select another song and write it either on the board or on paper, using as the beat unit a note which is different from the one in their books. For example:

Faith of Our Fathers (3/4)	Write in 3/2.
Old MacDonald (4/4)	Write in 4/8.
When Johnny Comes Marching Home (6/8)	Write in 6/16.
America (3/4)	Write in 3/8 and 3/2.

After this has been done the class should sing the different notations of the same song simultaneously. The fact that when these different notations are sung together they sound exactly the same impresses upon the pupils the parallelism of

171

the notations, namely that they are simply <u>different</u> ways of writing the same rhythms.

At this point there should be no discussion as to the necessity for using more than one kind of beat note in simple measures and more than one kind of beat note in compound measures. The fact remains that a great deal of music has been written using one or more of the less common beat notes. Hence it would seem that music education in our schools should provide pupils with an opportunity to become acquainted with music notations of this type and variety, and thus prepare them to read and interpret them correctly.

It should be pointed out to the pupils that since the half note (♩) also is often used as the beat note, it becomes in these cases the "walking" note, and hence

♩ ♩ ♩ ♩   are "running" notes,

♩. ♪♩. ♪   is the long-short or "skipping" rhythm,

𝅝   𝅝   are two-beat notes,

𝅝·   𝅝·   are three-beat notes, and

‖𝅝‖   is the four-beat note.

The pupils should then be given an opportunity to figure out the following when the eighth note (♪) is the beat note or "walking" note:

♪♪ or ♫   are "running" notes,

♪. ♪ or ♫.   is the "skipping" rhythm,

♩   ♩   are two-beat notes,

♩.   ♩.   are three-beat notes, and

♩   ♩   are four-beat notes.

Many songs are printed with a 3/4 measure signature which should be played and sung at a fast enough tempo so that pupils will feel <u>one</u> beat in a measure instead of three. Therefore the dotted half note (♩.) becomes the actual beat note, and

♩   ♩   is the long-short or "skipping" combination

♩ ♩ ♩   are "running" notes; and the two-beat notes

are written   ♩. | ♩.   or   ♩. | ♩ x   or   ♩. | ♩ x x

172

Attention needs to be called also to the fact that in many songs printed in 4/4 measure the beat note is actually the half note ($\half$), with two beats to the measure. There are also many examples of music in 2/4 measure which move so slowly that the measure feeling is actually quadruple: four beats to the measure, the eighth note ($\eighth$) being the beat note.

The teacher should at all times sing songs and play selections in a musical manner. The artistic interpretation and feeling of a musical composition, be it a child's song or a symphony, should always take precedence over any mathematical considerations of the signature, as far as determining the true measure of a composition is concerned.

Musicianship demands not that we think less, but that we feel more.

Bibliography

ANNETT, THOMAS. Music in the Rural School. The Boston Music Company, Boston, 1938. Chapter IV of this book is devoted to a brief discussion of controlled and creative rhythm and support of eurhythmics in the schools. The last part of the chapter includes singing games and folk dances. Chapter VII presents the writer's ideas on creative music procedures in the schools.

ARMITAGE, THERESA, et al. Our First Music. C. C. Birchard and Company, Boston, 1941. This teacher's book ("A Singing School Series"), for use in the primary grades, contains many songs and musical selections useful in rhythmic activities. The material is divided into twenty-four "units," which the progressive teacher also will find very helpful.

BEATTIE, JOHN W., et al. The American Singer Series, Book One. American Book Company, New York, 1944. This book contains much excellent material for rhythm work in the primary grades, together with helpful directions for the teacher.

COLEMAN, SATIS N. Creative Music for Children. G. P. Putnam's Sons, New York, 1922. "The Development of the Rhythmic Sense" is the title of Chapter V of this illuminating book. The author advances the idea that rhythm must first find expression through the body, and gives suggestions for such development.

COLEMAN, SATIS N. Your Child's Music. The John Day Company, New York, 1939. Special attention is called to Chapters V and XI ("Creative Experiences" and "Note Reading Experiences") of this worthwhile book for teachers of children. The author stresses the importance of much association and experience with music before the introduction of notation.

DAVISON, ARCHIBALD T. Music Education in America. Harper and Brothers, New York, 1926. In Chapter III, "Music Teaching in the Elementary Schools," the writer suggests that rhythm be taught separately, and that it must be learned through physical motion. The entire chapter will be of interest to the elementary grade music teacher.

DILLER, A., and PAGE, K. S. How to Teach the Rhythm Band. G. Schirmer, Inc., New York, 1930. A very helpful presentation of procedures which may be followed in carrying on rhythm-band activities.

DILLER, A., and PAGE, K. S. Pre-School Music Book. G. Schirmer, Inc., New York, 1936. This excellent book furnishes many action songs and music and suggestions for simple rhythmic activities. The music is easy to play.

DRIVER, ANN. Music and Movement. Oxford University Press, New York, 1936. An outstanding book defining the nature of rhythm and outlining its development. The writer presents a most helpful exposition of the subject for the private and public school music teacher.

DYKEMA, PETER W., and CUNDIFF, HANNAH M. New School Music Handbook. C. C. Birchard and Company, Boston, 1939. Note 41 of this helpful book for teachers of music is entitled "Definite Rhythmic Responses and Introduction to Music Reading." It contains discussions of the place and use of the rhythm band, and of the importance of large bodily movements in the development of a sense of rhythm. The chapter closes with a provocative list of questions and suggestions for additional readings.

LEARNING MUSIC THROUGH RHYTHM

FARNSWORTH, CHARLES HUBERT. Education Through Music. American Book Company, New York, 1909. In the first part of Chapter VI the author advances his belief that the first stage of awakening musical ideas is through work in rhythm.

FOX, LILLIAN MOHR, and HOPKINS, L. THOMAS. Creative School Music. Silver Burdett Company, New York, 1936. In Chapters VIII and IX of this fine text on creative experiences for the schoolroom the writers give some ideas which should prove very helpful to the teacher who wishes to introduce the creative element into the child's rhythmic experiences. The suggestions for the use of the toy orchestra or rhythm band are excellent.

GEHRKENS, KARL WILSON. Music in the Grade Schools. C. C. Birchard and Company, Boston, 1934. An advocate of modified eurhythmics in the schoolroom presents in Chapter X of this text his reasons for their inclusion in the regular music period. In Chapter XI he gives many practical suggestions for the use of the rhythm band.

GLENN, MABELLE. Music Activities and Practices in the Kindergarten and Elementary Grades. Ginn and Company, Boston, 1940. In this book, which serves also as a teacher's manual for use with the elementary grade music books of The World of Music series, Miss Glenn has outlined the application of her principles of music education through the use of specific music materials. The procedures suggested will repay careful study.

GLENN, MABELLE, et al. Play a Tune, The World of Music series. Ginn and Company, Boston, 1936. A superior collection of musical numbers especially selected for such rhythmic activities as phrasing, meter-sensing, rhythmics, and dramatization.

HUBBARD, GEORGE E. Music Teaching in the Elementary Grades. American Book Company, New York, 1934. Chapter III of this book is entitled "First-Grade Music" and includes the author's ideas on rhythm bands and eurhythmics.

HUGHES, DOROTHY. Rhythmic Games and Dances. American Book Company, New York, 1942. A collection of musical selections for games, dances, phrasing, experience in measure and rhythms. Suggestions for their use are included, as well as detailed dance directions.

KRONE, BEATRICE PERHAM. Music in the New School. Neil A. Kjos Music Company, Chicago, 1941. In Chapter VI of this stimulating book the writer stresses the importance of much free rhythmic interpretation of music heard, as opposed to the more formal responses of Dalcroze eurhythmics. The chapter closes with a suggested list of musical selections which have proved useful in this connection.

McCONATHY, OSBOURNE, et al. Music in Rural Education. Silver Burdett Company, New York, 1933. The contents of Chapter VII, "The Rhythm Band," and of Chapter VIII, "Rhythm Play," will prove helpful to teachers in search of suggestions for carrying on these musical experiences in the primary grades.

MURSELL, JAMES L., and GLENN, MABELLE. The Psychology of School Music Teaching. Silver Burdett Company, New York, 1938. In Chapter VII of this text is found the following statement: "Rhythm must be taught through muscular response. Unless this is done, it can never be taught properly." The ideas of these writers on rhythmic training should be given serious consideration by music teachers.

MURSELL, JAMES L. Music in American Schools. Silver Burdett Company, New York, 1943. Chapter VII of this stimulating book answers the following questions: "What is rhythm?" "How do we experience rhythm?" "What are some sound instructional devices and procedures in the teaching of rhythm?" This music educator's answers are worthy of careful study.

Music Education. National Society for the Study of Education, Thirty-Fifth Yearbook, Part II, Public School Publishing Company, Bloomington, Ill., 1936. In Chapter XIII of this yearbook Dr. Will Earhart, director of music in the Pittsburgh schools, writes on creative activities in the school music program. His "Standards" and "Summary" are thought-provoking.

Music Education. National Society for the Study of Education, Thirty-Fifth Yearbook, Part II, Public School Publishing Company, Bloomington, Ill., 1936. Chapter VI of this yearbook was written by Mabelle Glenn, director of music in the Kansas City schools, probably the leading exponent of the importance of developing the rhythmic sense of the child. In this article she outlines her beliefs and practices in the furnishing of experiences in rhythm. In Chapter XVII of this volume will be found suggestions by Miss Hood for teaching music in a small rural school. A special section is devoted to the work in rhythm.

Music Education in the Elementary School. California State Department of Education, Sacramento, 1939. This outstanding course of study in elementary-school music includes many suggestions for the treatment of rhythm in relation to the music education of the child. A perusal of the table of contents will reveal the pages upon which may be found directions for the conduct of rhythmic activities.

NORTON, ALMA M. Teaching School Music. C. C. Crawford, Los Angeles, 1932. Miss Norton stresses the importance of pre-experience in rhythm before the study of music notation is begun. Chapter II, on furnishing pre-experience of all sorts in music, touches on a fundamental aspect of music education.

PENNINGTON, JO. The Importance of Being Rhythmic. G. P. Putnam's Sons, New York, 1925. An indispensable text for musician and educator, who will find the author's presentation vital and practical.

RENSTROM, MOISELLE. Musical Adventures. Deseret Book Company, Salt Lake City, 1943. A very valuable collection for use in creative dramatization in the primary grades. The piano arrangements are quite easy.

RENSTROM, MOISELLE. Rhythm Fun for Little Folks. Pioneer Music Press, Salt Lake City, 1944. The teacher of kindergarten and primary grades will find this collection to be an excellent source of easy and effective materials.

RILEY, ALICE C. D., GAYNOR, JESSIE L., and BLAKE, DOROTHY GAYNOR. Thirty Rhythmic Pantomimes. The John Church Company, Philadelphia, 1937. This publication outlines some splendid rhythmic activities, with music, for free and suggestive interpretation suitable for use in the primary grades.

SURETTE, THOMAS WHITNEY. Music and Life. Houghton Mifflin Company, Boston, 1917. Chapter III of this book is devoted to a discussion of public-school music. Included in the chapter is a discussion of the author's statement "The arithmetical complications of rhythm in music should never be taught to young children at all."

THORN, ALICE. Music for Young Children. Charles Scribner's Sons, New York, 1929. A most valuable book for teachers of pre-school and primary grade children. The suggestions for rhythmic activities are especially good.

LEARNING MUSIC THROUGH RHYTHM

TOBITT, JANET, and WHITE, ALICE. Dramatized Ballads. E. P. Dutton and
Company, New York, 1937. This publication contains many folk songs with
suggestions for rhythmic dramatizations, and is especially designed for upper
grades and adults.

Alphabetical Index of Music

*After a title indicates it is an instrumental composition.

PRINTED IN THE UNITED STATES OF AMERICA